"Feeding my child turned out to be more stressful than I ever expected, and Solid Starts offers the most comprehensive, practical advice out there."
—Myleik Teele, life coach and community curator

"Every new parent will benefit from this essential read. It provides clear guidance that supports both the baby and the family, paving the way for positive, enjoyable eating experiences and a healthy long-term relationship with food."
—Sumner Brooks, MPH, RDN, co-author of
How to Raise an Intuitive Eater

"*Solid Starts for Babies* offers evidence-based information on food allergies and allergen introduction in an easy-to-digest and reassuring format, helping families overcome fear and take action to reduce food allergy risk."
—Ruchi Gupta, MD, MPH, professor of pediatrics at Northwestern University Feinberg School of Medicine and author of *Food Without Fear*

"*Solid Starts for Babies* is an invaluable resource for parents who want an evidence-based and balanced approach to introducing solids. The book's expert insights into self-feeding bring a refreshing depth that's hard to find in the crowded field of parenting advice."
—Dr. Ashley Lerman, DDS

"A thorough, must-read guide for parents who want to nourish and nurture their baby's health and happiness while they learn to eat."
—Jill Castle, MS, RDN, founder of The Nourished Child and author of
Kids Thrive at Every Size and *Fearless Feeding*

"*Solid Starts for Babies* guides parents in introducing a variety of foods, including commonly allergenic foods, with the goal of nurturing joyful eating habits and reducing the risk of food allergy."
—Marion Groetch, MS, RD, associate professor, Icahn School of Medicine at Mount Sinai and co-editor of *Health Professional's Guide to Nutrition Management of Food Allergies*

"When parents ask me infant feeding questions, Solid Starts is always my first recommendation. With this book, I'm thrilled parents will find the information they need quickly and comprehensively from a team of pediatric professionals who truly care about the well-being of the whole family at mealtimes."

—Mallory Whitmore, MEd, @theformulamom

"*Solid Starts for Babies* is the book every parent needs for learning to feed their babies to grow into independent and healthy eaters. This evidence-based guide walks parents through not just the practical steps of introducing foods, but also how to navigate common challenges when doing so. This is the new must-have book for parents and babies."

—Dr. Sara Reardon, founder of @the.vagina.whisperer and mom of two

SOLID STARTS
FOR BABIES

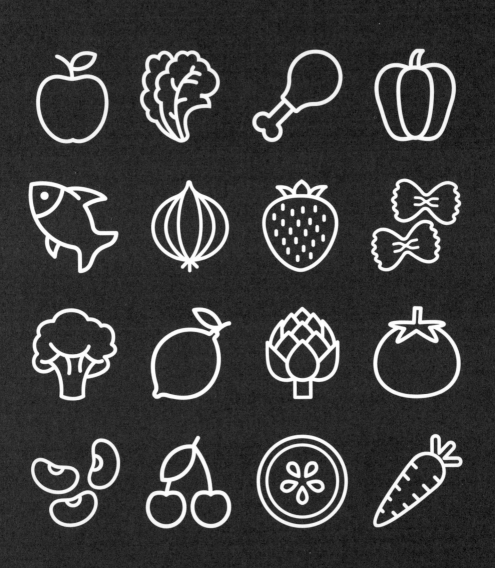

SOLID STARTS
— FOR BABIES —

How to Introduce Solid Food
and Raise a Happy Eater

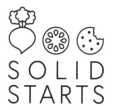

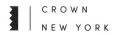

CROWN
NEW YORK

CROWN

An imprint of the Crown Publishing Group
A division of Penguin Random House LLC
crownpublishing.com

Illustrations by Carmen Deñó (chapter openers/spots),
Lucy Anderson (infographics/charts), and Todd Detwiler (anatomical).

Library of Congress Cataloging-in-Publication Data
Names: Best, Jenny, editor. | Solid Starts (Firm), author. Title: Solid starts for babies : how to introduce solid food and raise a happy eater / Solid Starts. Description: First edition. | New York : Crown, [2025] | Identifiers: LCCN 2024051477 | ISBN 9780593735411 (Hardcover) | ISBN 9780593735435 (trade paperback) | ISBN 9780593735428 (ebook) Subjects: LCSH: Baby foods. | Infants—Nutrition. | Infants—Weaning. Classification: LCC RJ216 .S5655 2025 | DDC 641.5/6222—dc23/eng/20241115
LC record available at https://lccn.loc.gov/2024051477

Hardcover ISBN 978-0-593-73541-1
Ebook ISBN 978-0-593-73542-8

Editor: Libby Burton
Editorial assistants: Cierra Hinckson and Brittney Bailey
Production editor: Ashley Pierce
Text designer: Andrea Lau
Production manager: Heather Williamson
Copyeditor: Amy J. Schneider
Proofreaders: Sigi Nacson and Miriam Taveras
Indexer: Ken DellaPenta
Publicist: Tammy Blake
Marketer: Chantelle Walker

Manufactured in the United States of America

1st Printing

First Edition

For those who have been pressured to eat or
forced to finish their plate.

And for all the children to come.

May they find their love for food on their own terms.

Contents

About the Authors

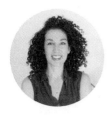

Kary Rappaport
OTR/L, MS, SCFES, IBCLC
Pediatric Feeding/Swallowing Specialist

Kary Rappaport is a licensed pediatric occupational therapist, certified feeding and swallowing specialist, and international board-certified lactation consultant based in Oregon.

For nearly twenty years, Kary has supported families with evaluation and treatment of feeding and swallowing challenges in infants and young children. She has extensive training and experience including administering modified barium swallow studies for this age group, managing complex feeding issues, and developing protocols and feeding programs. Kary has practiced as a pediatric occupational therapist in a variety of settings, including in-home, outpatient clinics, pediatric primary care offices, dental clinics, and leading medical institutions, including Children's Hospital Los Angeles.

As a mom of two young children, Kary is a passionate advocate for clinical care that improves family access to connection-driven and research-supported interventions with infant feeding, from birth to solid food to family meals. Throughout her career she has trained medical professionals and developed continuing education programs in infant feeding and swallowing in a wide range of clinical settings. In partnership with Kimberly Grenawitzke, she co-created professional courses on pediatric feeding which have influenced pediatric clinical care at numerous pediatric hospitals, university programs, and therapy clinics in the United States. Kary continues to teach and mentor fellow pediatric professionals through her leadership of Solid Starts PRO—an international network of medical professionals who are supporting parents with raising happy eaters.

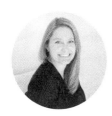

Kimberly Grenawitzke
OTD, OTR/L, SCFES, IBCLC, CNT
Pediatric Feeding/Swallowing Specialist

Kimberly Grenawitzke is a licensed pediatric occupational therapist with specialty certification in feeding, eating, and swallowing; an international board-certified lactation consultant; and certified neonatal therapist based in Michigan.

Kim supports families with evaluation and treatment of feeding and swallowing challenges in infants and young children, including those with extreme prematurity, cancer/blood disorders, congenital heart disease, and other health conditions. For more than fifteen years, she has worked in both home settings and leading medical institutions, including Children's Hospital Los Angeles and Lucile Packard Children's Hospital Stanford. Kim earned her doctorate of occupational therapy from the University of Southern California.

As a mom of two young children, Kim is a passionate advocate for research and education that helps bridge the gap between pediatric healthcare and a family's journey with infant feeding, from birth to solid food to family meals. She has created numerous continuing education opportunities to guide medical professionals, including the first doctoral residency program in occupational therapy at Children's Hospital Los Angeles. In partnership with Kary Rappaport, she co-created professional courses on pediatric feeding for clinical training programs at Stanford University, the University of Southern California, California Children's Services, and numerous pediatric therapy clinics in the United States. Their courses serve as the foundation for Solid Starts PRO and its pediatric community around the world.

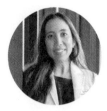

Dr. Rachel Ruiz

MD, FAAP, CLC

Pediatrician and Pediatric Gastroenterologist

Dr. Rachel Ruiz is a board-certified pediatrician and pediatric gastroenterologist. She is based in California, where she serves as an attending pediatric gastroenterologist at Santa Clara Valley Medical Center and an affiliated clinical instructor of pediatric gastroenterology at Lucile Packard Children's Hospital Stanford. Prior to her current roles, Dr. Ruiz completed her pediatric gastroenterology fellowship at Lucile Packard Children's Hospital Stanford. She is also a fellow of the American Academy of Pediatrics, certified lactation counselor, and a member of the North American Society for Pediatric Gastroenterology, Hepatology & Nutrition. She earned her doctorate of medicine from Vanderbilt University School of Medicine, and subsequently completed her pediatric residency at Monroe Carell Jr. Children's Hospital at Vanderbilt.

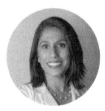

Dr. Sakina Bajowala

MD, FAAAAI

Pediatric Allergist/Immunologist

Dr. Sakina Bajowala is a board-certified allergist and immunologist and an internationally recognized expert in the treatment of life-threatening food allergies. Based in Illinois, she is the medical director of Kaneland Allergy & Asthma Center and executive director of the Kaneland Food Allergy Foundation. After earning her doctorate of medicine from Rush Medical College, she completed her pediatric residency at Comer Children's Hospital of the University of Chicago and her allergy and clinical immunology fellowship at Rush University Medical Center. Dr. Bajowala is an active member of the American Academy of Allergy, Asthma, and Immunology; the American College of Allergy, Asthma, and Immunology; and the Illinois Society of Allergy, Asthma, and Immunology, of which she is currently serving as president.

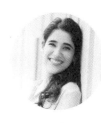

Venus S. Kalami
MNSP, RD, CSP
Pediatric Dietitian/Nutritionist

Venus Kalami is a registered dietitian and board-certified specialist in pediatric nutrition with specializations in digestive health and food allergy nutrition, based in California. With more than ten years of health experience, she has worked primarily at leading hospitals, including Stanford Medicine Children's Health. Her expertise covers infant and toddler nutrition, general pediatrics, and children with medical complexities. She completed her dietitian training at Stanford Medicine and earned her master's degree in nutrition science and policy from Tufts University. At Stanford Medicine Children's Health, she established inaugural nutrition programs for the nationally recognized pediatric inflammatory bowel disease and celiac disease centers of excellence. She has published research on psychosocially informed nutrition, spoken nationally on cultural diversity in infant feeding, and led continuing education to thousands of health professionals.

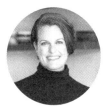

Jenny Best
Founder

Jenny is a mom of three on a quest to help families find joy at the table. Passionate about food and food culture, Jenny founded Solid Starts to make it easier for parents to learn how to introduce any food to their baby. Jenny is the creator of the award-winning First Foods® database, a searchable inventory of 400+ foods with step-by-step instructions, how-to videos, practical strategies, and recipes within the Solid Starts App.

Introduction

When my twins turned 6 months old, I held a chicken drumstick in front of each baby. They were panting for it, reaching for it. Their feet were kicking with excitement as each of them snatched one out of my hand and brought it right to their mouths. I stepped back, stunned. Could it really be this easy to get a baby to eat? This natural? I couldn't believe my eyes. We had followed traditional recommendations and spoon-fed our first child, and the experience had been so different. As I watched the twins happily munch on their food—without needing any help from me—questions started to build . . . If letting a baby feed themself was so obviously natural, why weren't more pediatricians talking about it?

—Jenny Best, founder, Solid Starts

The face of a baby who has been given a taste of something they find delicious is a beautiful thing to see. Equally hilarious are the expressions that pop up when they encounter a food that they find sour or bitter or just plain confusing. A few tastes later, you can see it dawn that they might actually like it. Or they will fling it onto the floor, which, from baby's point of view, is a perfectly reasonable response.

Teaching a baby to eat solid food can be a slow and steady process. Set a pace that feels right for both you and baby. Babies need lots of time and practice to build the skills to eat real food, and together you will learn so much along the way. When should you begin? As you'll learn, most babies can be offered real food around 6 months of age, when they have the strength to sit upright, and the skills to coordinate the many movements needed for bringing food to the mouth and swallowing it. This developmental moment tips off an incredible window in baby's life, a magical time when they are simultaneously eager to explore things with their mouth, easily interested in new foods, and have key physiological reflexes that help them learn how to chew. This magic window is a biological wonder of development, and by the end of this book, you'll know everything you need to support baby as they learn how to feed themself.

Our approach is based on the idea that baby can eat the same food that you do. That giving baby the foods and flavors you enjoy from the start lays a strong foundation from which they can explore. This approach not only makes it possible to make one meal for everyone in the family, it also enables baby to learn by watching you eat the same food, which is exactly what their brain is set up to do.

Welcome to the Baby Food Revolution

Solid Starts was created with the idea that things could be different. We set out to challenge the status quo and change the conversation, and we are so happy to have you here with us, being curious, doing the research, asking big questions. Our mission has always been, and continues to be, to help parents raise children who love to eat and who listen to their bodies.

A wealth of new research shows there are tangible benefits for babies who are allowed to practice feeding themselves as soon as they are ready to start solids and that it's safe to do so. However, much of the well-known literature is woefully outdated, and many health institutions and governmental bodies are late to the conversation. There is a popularized notion that babies *need* special baby food, when in fact it's simply not true.

What if we were to tell you that baby food itself is a commercial invention? That, in reality, almost any food can be made safe for babies? What if we were to tell you that many commercial baby foods don't even contain the nutrients that babies need? Or that there's no developmental necessity to start with a thin puree and graduate to a thicker mash? That much of what we as parents have been historically told about infant feeding are myths and fallacies?

What if we focused less on tricking baby to open their mouth for the spoon or how much puree baby swallows and more on the joy of eating? What if you had the knowledge to start solids more flexibly, in a way that works for your unique family? What if we trusted our babies to know when they are full? How might our babies benefit if we focused not on bites taken but on the child's relationship with food?

If you want to raise a child who has a positive relationship with food, who trusts themself, who trusts you, and who eagerly tries new things, you're in the right place. We want to give you the information you need to feel safe and confident to let baby eat enthusiastically on their own. When you give baby the space to explore and fumble, they develop skills that are highly transferable, helping them grow up to be more adaptable and independent—at the table and beyond.

The Solid Starts Team

Our team is composed of pediatric professionals: a board-certified pediatrician and pediatric gastroenterologist, licensed feeding therapists and infant swallowing specialists, a board-certified dietitian/nutritionist, and a board-certified allergist/immunologist. We have deliberately created an integrative team, giving ourselves an opportunity to step out of our silos and create something useful that covers all of the bases for parents and professionals.

Our approach stems from the work of Gill Rapley, PhD who coined and defined the concept of baby-led weaning, and of

Kary Rappaport and Kim Grenawitzke, two occupational thera-pists with deep expertise in pediatric feeding and lactation who have worked to encourage infant self-feeding in various hospi-tals to help medically complex babies more quickly develop oral motor skills and form positive relationships with food.[1] Together, Kim and Kary have become mentors to thousands of pediatric professionals around the world. They are truly the leading minds in infant feeding and possess deep expertise in food refusal at all ages. Their insight and wisdom is woven throughout every sentence in this book.

Our team also includes Dr. Rachel Ruiz, a double-board-certified pediatrician and pediatric gastroenterologist and clini-cal instructor at Lucile Packard Children's Hospital at Stanford, and she isn't afraid to question the norms in medicine. Among the first pediatricians to publicly endorse the idea of letting babies feed themselves, Dr. Ruiz combs through research and often pokes holes in it. Together, we discovered a number of flaws in how the U.S. government collects data on choking and how the flawed data has been misinterpreted and reported over the years by various publications and media outlets, leading to a fear of choking that, quite simply, is out of proportion with the statisti-cal likelihood of it occurring.

Our recommendations on allergens come from Dr. Sakina Bajowala, a leading physician in pediatric food allergy preven-tion and treatment and the author of her own book, *The Food Allergy Fix.* Whereas many healthcare providers are overrestrict-ing foods to their patients, cutting them off from ever possibly tol-erating those foods, Dr. B is an advocate for dietary diversity and is at the forefront of rapidly evolving treatments for food allergy, including sublingual and oral immunotherapies, which can help individuals safely expand their diets, decrease the likelihood of allergic reactions, and improve their quality of life.

When it comes to nutrition, we take a real-life approach thanks to Venus Kalami, our board-certified pediatric dietitian and nutritionist with a passion for making infant self-feeding realistic and accessible for all. She has published in reputable journals and presented nationally on the importance of psycho-socially informed, culturally sensitive, and weight-inclusive nutrition. Her goal is to help families trust themselves to nourish their baby's (and their own) relationship with food and their body.

The inspiration for Solid Starts came from my lived experience, but our work today represents the team's collective expertise and desire to help future families. —Jenny Best

The evidence for our approach is woven throughout this book. We have tried, diligently, to shine a light on existing literature, acknowledge where more research is needed, and highlight often-overlooked studies and findings. But the real proof is all around us. It's in the parents who have chosen to let their babies feed themselves and who have watched their babies grow into toddlers who love to eat. It's in the growing community of pediatric professionals who are empowering their patients to share the foods they love with their babies. And it's in people like you who are taking the time to learn more and challenge the status quo.

We have served nearly 20 million parents in every single country of the world. Here are a couple of messages from them, which we share so that you might feel less alone:

"When my relationship with Solid Starts began, it took a long time, a lot of patience, a lot of listening to my child and his cues, but we're making real progress. We have been going through recipes, trying new foods, having new experiences. He is really starting to enjoy food and it's because of Solid Starts."

"Solid Starts has completely revamped motherhood for me. It has been a major part of my healing process with post-partum depression and regaining a purpose with my baby . . . it gave me confidence and helped me take care of our son."

"I was so scared to feed solid food to my daughter. I just had so much anxiety around wanting to make sure she has a healthy relationship with food as I definitely never have. Watching my daughter become confident with feeding herself and enjoying food just makes me overwhelmingly happy. I cannot thank you enough for making me feel comfortable and giving me the confidence to help teach my daughter how to eat and help her enjoy it as well."

How to Use This Book

We wrote *Solid Starts for Babies* for parents, expecting parents, and caregivers, as well as pediatric professionals, to share the message that when baby is ready to begin the transition from breast or bottle to solid food, baby can enjoy almost any food with some basic safety modifications.

Keep in mind that we are never trying to prescribe specific foods for baby. We don't want you to get in the habit of making special, separate meals for your children, now or later. In fact, quite the opposite. The best thing you can do is bring baby into your unique food culture right away.

In **Part 1, Exploring Solids,** you'll get a run-through on why letting baby feed themself is an investment in the future, learn about the evidence, wonder at the myth of baby food, and marvel at nature's wisdom and the biological underpinnings behind why we start solids around 6 months of age.

Part 2, Building Trust, explores the connection between mealtimes, our relationship with baby, and baby's relationship with their own body. You'll learn about responsive feeding, which takes into account baby's engagement, and can help baby learn, grow, and work through new challenges. You'll also learn all about baby's biology, and the reflexes that help prevent choking as they learn to eat.

Part 3, Building Skill, gets right into it, from when to start to what equipment you need, before doing a deep dive into how to choose first foods and how to prep the food by age, prepare for the expected (and unexpected), and get baby involved with cups and other utensils.

Part 4, Building Resilience, gets into the basics of hunger and fullness cues, covers baby nutrition, and demystifies growth and weight charts. It also is of special importance, because research about when to start common allergens has evolved a great deal in the past years. Specifically, it is now understood that there are preventive benefits to introducing peanuts, milk, eggs, and more as soon as baby is developmentally ready for solids (and in some cases, earlier). We've got you covered with clear guidance as to what, when, and how, including detailed allergen introduction schedules.

Part 5, Feeders and Growers, introduces you to various ways to engage baby, as well as offers insights into how they grow and learn at each stage, so you can learn to help them help themself.

And yes, there's more, because when it comes to teaching baby to eat, there are always more questions, and we have answers. We will walk you through what to do about common mealtime challenges such as overstuffing, gagging, and food refusal to reflux.

We hear from so many parents who rely on scraps of information from various incomplete sources, much of it outdated and counterproductive. You deserve better and so do your kids. That's why we built our app and wrote this book: to give you a thoughtful and useful resource that you can rely on again and again, from that first high chair moment to toddlerhood. Use the resources together. Download our app to access our award-winning First Foods database, and keep the book handy for a deeper dive.

We hope this book inspires you to find joy in sharing food with baby and helps you trust them at the table. Give baby space to explore, fumble, and learn. Trust that the foods you love to eat can be made safe for baby. Trust that baby knows when they are hungry or full. Trust that even if you feel nervous to start, with each day both you and baby will grow more confident. And on days when it feels like everything is falling apart, trust that you can always start fresh tomorrow.

Disclaimer

As you read, please keep in mind that this book contains general feeding information that is informed by typical infant development.

The guidance we provide is geared toward children who are typically developing, healthy, and growing as expected by their medical team. Because all babies and families are unique, we expect that some of this information will not apply or will require modification. If your baby is following a different developmental pathway than expected, or if they have a disability or any medical needs, this information will likely need to be adapted. The guidelines found in this book can often be easily adapted to your unique child's needs in collaboration with your child's healthcare team.

For children with restricted diets or food allergies, suggested foods may be substituted for ones that are appropriate for baby. For example, a baby with a milk allergy could try a coconut-based yogurt in place of cow's-milk yogurt. Children who have restricted diets, food allergies, and medical conditions that affect their growth and nutrition (such as cystic fibrosis, heart conditions, and digestive conditions) may need nutritional supplements, specialized formulas, and closer support with feeding and nutrition from pediatric specialists.

Many children with developmental delays, disabilities, sensory differences, or medical complexity will need more time and support to build a sense of comfort, safety, and skill with solid foods. If your baby has had any past negative experiences involving their face or mouth (such as intubation, feeding tubes, or cleft lip/palate) or difficulty with breathing (needing any amount of oxygen support), they may need more patience and even more positive food experiences than usual before they gain confidence. Past history of food allergies, pain associated with eating, or even fear around food can all impact the pace of this transition and how much you can push baby when it comes to learning new skills at the table. Even when the stakes feel high, it is important to honor your child's needs, autonomy, and willingness to engage in mealtimes. Every child has their own starting point and progresses on their own timeline. Use this book but also check in frequently with your healthcare team to be sure your child's unique needs are being met. You can also check out *Your Baby Can Self-Feed, Too: Adapted Baby-Led Weaning for Children with Developmental Delays or Other Feeding Challenges,* an excellent resource to help guide you through adapting baby's solid food journey as necessary.

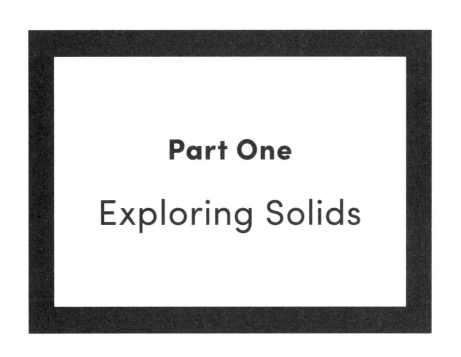

Part One

Exploring Solids

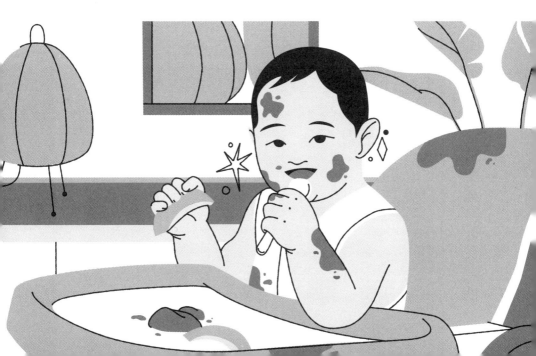

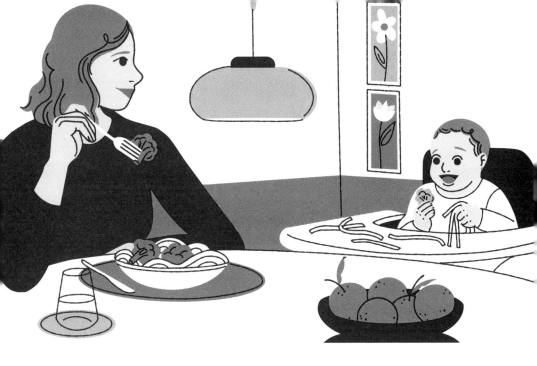

Chapter One

Choosing the Long Game

Y ou sit down with your baby for dinner. You're having a simple meal tonight, something that was easy to prepare, which you enjoy. You serve your baby the same food you serve yourself. There's no pressure to eat anything. You happily focus on your meal, enjoying your food while baby smashes and explores theirs. You converse with your baby even though you're not sure they understand you. Laughter fills the room. You are relaxed and calm. Everyone eats what they want, and leaves what they don't, including baby, who pushes food off the table to let you know they are done. There's food all over baby's face, and you laugh about that, too.

Human beings are connection-driven creatures. There is a special feeling of ease and comfort when we are doing things alongside other people we love. Mealtimes are just as much about personal connections as they are about the food. This is true for baby, too. Eating with you is a space for developing relationships as much as eating skills. The preceding anecdote isn't really about dinner. It's a story about relationships: the relationship between baby and their food, between baby and their body, and between you and baby. Every meal has potential to strengthen each of these connections.

It may sound obvious to say that love and trust are essential in all this, but sometimes what is most basic is what bears the most repeating. Parents and caregivers want to feed babies in the best way they can, but even the most attentive feeder can fall into the trap of focusing so deeply on the details of *what* to feed baby (or how much baby consumes) that they lose sight of the big picture—the joy of food and connection at the table.

When you make the table a place of connection, where everyone feels safe, cared for, and listened to, your child will want to keep coming back. They will feel seen and ready to learn. They will understand what it means to feel full in a way that is self-determined. Focusing on your relationship with your baby at the table is what we like to call the long game—where all of our micro decisions at meals build the future and the child's long-term relationship with food, the table, and you.

The opposite of the long game is the short game: counting bites. Fretting over the number of milligrams of this or that your baby is eating. Distracting baby so they will open their mouth for one more spoonful. All of this detracts from what is important: creating a dynamic where baby is ready and wanting to learn how to eat.

Creating a Space for Connection

The first step in baby's journey of learning to eat is interest. The key to getting baby interested and excited to explore food is their connection with the person who is eating with them.

As we will discuss in Chapter 4, connection is a basic human need. When baby is in connection with you, they want to be near you and watch you. When a baby is connected to a loving caregiver, they naturally imitate them and more easily learn from them. Babies have all the necessary tools to safely learn to eat, and in the majority of cases, these skills will naturally present themselves when baby has a strong relationship with a caregiver at the table.

Throughout this book we'll give you examples of what it looks like to create a mealtime space where baby wants to be. We'll help you understand what your role is and how to stay in connection with baby throughout this process. By the time you're done reading, you'll understand why so many people are choosing to let their babies self-feed, how it will benefit baby, when to start, what you'll need—and how to implement these ideas starting on day one.

We'll also get into all of the details—the gear, the foods, and how you prepare them—because details matter, but only if baby is ready and willing to be at the table.

It's very hard to make a baby eat when they don't want to. You can create the right conditions to interest them in a meal, but ultimately, a child must choose to eat. To do this, they need to choose to pick up a utensil or piece of food, open their mouth, and accept the food. Any attempt to get them to eat when they don't want to will backfire, which research shows can negatively impact their relationship with food—and their relationship with you.[1]

Mealtimes happen multiple times a day, every day, making them a unique opportunity to establish and reinforce tangible skills like using a fork, chewing, and drinking from a straw, but also important intangible skills like handling disappointment, self-sufficiency, problem solving, and self-regulation. The adults at the table are learning too—to gradually let go and trust baby. Baby and caregiver are learning to trust each other.

This is why we begin our book here and will return to this idea of connection at the table. Everything else follows from there.

Investing in the Long Game Will Pay Off

Teaching babies to eat solid food isn't just about how much they eat in that moment; it's about how you hope that the child will come to view food and meals in the weeks and years after. That's the long game. For some, this hope might look like a child who enjoys eating, loves coming to the table with you, and has a positive relationship with food and their body. For others it might look like a child who is highly adaptable at meals, willing to try new foods and flavors. These are long-game goals.

The short game, in contrast, focuses on the here and now. It is heavily dependent on how your day is going. It's more about what we need to do minute to minute to get through a certain moment than what we are working toward ultimately. In the ideal world, our short-game choices would perfectly line up with and support our long-game aspirations, but more often than not, immediate needs get in the way.

For some, the short-game decisions might look like spoon-feeding baby to minimize the mess so they can get out the door on time. For others it might look like letting a toddler watch TV to keep the peace at dinner. Or only serving favorite snack foods to avoid tantrums. In a short-game moment—whatever that moment may be—by all means, do what you need to do. You can always try again.

If baby is approaching 6 months of age, now is a terrific time to consider your mealtime goals and start creating the patterns and practices that will get you there. If eating dinner together is something you want, start now. If you want baby to love foods that are culturally important to you, share those dishes early on. While it may seem easier to wait to start these things, a unique window in time is about to open, where baby is incredibly receptive to new foods and practices. In other words, it's easier to teach baby this now than it will be later when they are a toddler.

After 12 months of age, many toddlers develop a natural resistance to trying new foods. This new phase is labeled "toddler neophobia" by some researchers, because it appears to be a significant fear of trying new things, including foods. And after baby's first birthday it is often harder—not easier—to teach a toddler how to chew foods and enjoy new flavors. Not only is it harder to teach a child to chew when they will not put the food in their mouth, but also key physiological reflexes that help babies easily learn these skills fade with age. Does that mean the child who starts late will never learn? Of course not. But when it comes to food, it's simply easier to teach many of these skills when a baby is younger. Is it a guarantee that your toddler will eat everything they were served as a baby? Unfortunately, no. But the research is clear: the more exposure a baby gets to a wide variety of foods, the more likely it is they will continue to eat them (or eventually come back to them) in toddlerhood and beyond.[2,3,4]

To build new skills, babies need lots of time and space for repetitive practice. The same goes for eating. The more you spoon-feed a baby, the longer it will take for them to learn how to feed themselves. Similarly, the more you rely on commercially designated baby foods, the longer it will take that child to accept the foods the rest of the family is eating. Yes, pouches and puffs can have a role to play in the short game. Please, use them when you need them. Just keep the long game in mind.

When we prioritize the long game and let babies fumble their way through, we provide children with important learning opportunities. On a macro scale, we want baby to learn that they are capable of learning new things and handling challenges. On a micro scale, we want baby to learn basic skills like self-feeding and chewing thoroughly. The more you get out of the way and let baby practice by trial and error, the faster they will learn—and that's a long game that benefits parents and children alike.

Choosing Joy

Our approach is designed to help you foster a child's inherent motivation around food. With this in mind, we invite you to let go of any feeding rules and requirements that may have been passed down to you. Let go of any desire to achieve perfection. Skip suggestions that do not seem to fit your baby's or family's needs. Release rigidity to make space for something much more important: joy. There is no perfect meal. There is no perfect food. There is no perfect high chair, plate, or utensil. But there is an ideal environment to learn. And that's a joyful one.

If you want to support baby's journey toward becoming a child who listens to their body and trusts their hunger and fullness cues, who feels at ease around food, and who loves eating with you, make the table a place they want to be. Focus on connection, on sharing the foods you love, and trusting that baby can do it. The rest will naturally follow.

Summary

✓ Babies learn best when they feel connected to (and trust) their caregiver.

✓ Babies learn to eat by watching you eat the same food.

✓ Consider your mealtime goals and hopes for your child and how you want to get there.

✓ Baby is most receptive to new foods and practices before 12 months of age.

✓ After their first birthday, many toddlers develop a resistance to trying new foods.

✓ When you make the table a place of connection, your child will want to come back.

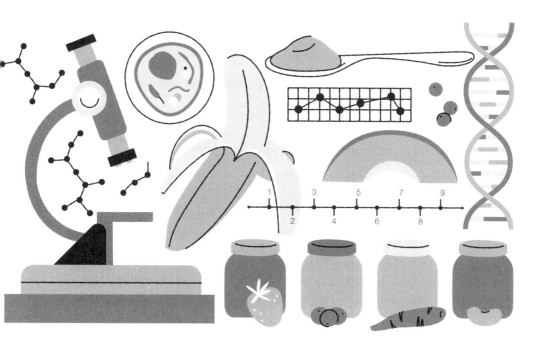

Chapter Two

Evolving with the Evidence

The wet-nurse may take a moderate quantity of sound porter, or of mild (but not old or strong) ale, with her dinner. Tea should be taken at half-past five or six o'clock; supper at nine, which should consist of a slice or two of cold meat, or of cheese if she prefer it, with half a pint of porter or mild ale: occasionally, a basin of gruel may be substituted, with advantage. Hot and late suppers are, prejudicial to the mother, or wet-nurse, and, consequently, to the child. The wet-nurse must be in bed every night by ten o'clock.

—*Advice to a Young Mother on the Management of Her Children* by Pye Henry Chavasse, 1865

Advice on how to care for babies can come with some very loud voices and some very strong opinions. With every generation, many of those ideas (thankfully) change. At Solid Starts, we believe in following the evidence, and, where evidence is lacking, to lean on the science of physiology and child development. Let's take a look back to see what people used to think, why things changed, and how we arrived from the myths of the past to the science-backed practices we recommend in these pages.

We begin our tour in the 1800s. You're a new mother, and for the first year of baby's life, all they will get is breast milk, with wet nurses' help to make this possible. Solid food won't be offered until baby is around a year old.

Fast forward to the 1950s, when the popular magazines of the day are full of images of jolly infants being spoon-fed from little glass jars. When your doctor tells you that your 1-month-old infant is ready to start commercial baby food, you do what they suggest. After all, the food is made by men in white coats, "scientifically" concocted.

Now jump to the 1980s. You see an ad in a magazine suggesting that your breast milk may not be enough, and that you should supplement with commercial baby food. At the same time, you are advised to start solids around 4 months of age but to avoid serving baby allergens like egg and peanut until they are 3 years old.

And now here we are in the mid-2020s, in an era when pediatric authorities generally agree that the optimal time to introduce solids is around 6 months of age or when a baby shows developmental readiness. And because we saw allergies in the pediatric population surge alongside the old recommendations, doctors today (should) know that we need to introduce common allergens like egg and peanut right away when starting solids, if not earlier.

Over the years, as medical professionals have learned more about infant nutrition, allergy, immunology, and child development, how and when we introduce solid food to babies has drastically changed.

Alongside these changes in the medical community, we've seen a shift in how we choose to parent and interact with children. So if you find yourself in disagreement with your parents, grandparents, or in-laws about how to feed baby, you're not alone. You may even get differing opinions from different doctors and health professionals. Research has rapidly evolved and it's difficult to keep up.

Age of Introducing Solids Over Time

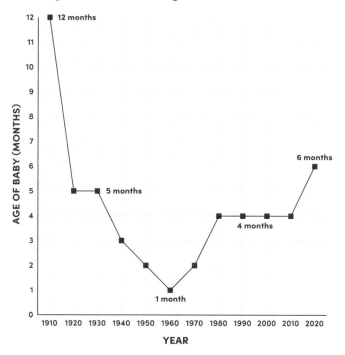

Building on research by New York University professor Amy Bentley, this line graph demonstrates how the age of introduction of solid food has varied widely over time. In instances of wide variation, such as the 1950s and 1960s, the lowest commonly recommended age was plotted. Research and pediatrics have advanced since the late nineteenth century. Today most leading pediatric authorities agree: around 6 months of age is ideal for introducing solid food.

Today's evidence shows us that when babies are exposed to a wide variety of colorful foods, tastes, and textures—before 12 months of age—they are more likely to be open to exploring new foods later on.[1] We also know that there is a key age window in infancy in which a baby most easily—and safely—learns how to chew.[2,3] And after decades of watching food allergies rise, there is now compelling evidence that early and sustained exposure to allergens can actually decrease the likelihood that the child will develop allergies to these foods altogether.[4,5,6]

It can be startling to learn how long it can take for healthcare institutions to change recommendations, even in the face of strong evidence. One study showed that it can take up to seventeen years for new research to be translated into a broad change in care recommendations within the healthcare community.[7]

Today, as we write, the most current research says:

→ The best time to introduce solid food is when a baby shows developmental signs of readiness, usually around 6 months of age.[8]

→ Just about any food your family enjoys can be made safe for baby once they are developmentally ready to start solids.[9]

→ Healthy, typically developing babies don't need baby food for nutrition or to learn how to eat solid food.[10]

→ Babies do not need to progress through stages of gradual thickness of foods, as commercially prepared baby food advertises. It's not necessary and it isn't a very effective way for most babies to learn to chew.[11]

→ Teeth aren't needed for baby to break down most foods, and baby's chewing skills won't just appear when baby has reached a certain age or sprouted a certain number of teeth. Babies are born with reflexes to help them learn how to chew.[12,13]

→ Introducing common allergens like egg and peanut as soon as baby is ready for solids and then serving them at least one to two times per week throughout the toddler years helps prevent allergies to these foods from developing altogether.[14,15]

→ The more tastes, textures, and foods a baby is exposed to before 12 months of age, the more likely it is that they will be open to new foods as toddlers and beyond.[16]

While the research isn't perfect, it's a start—and a much stronger one than the absolute lack of research that supported the entire industry of baby food—more to come on this shortly. We expect continued investigation of these themes over the next ten years. The bottom line is that specially pureed baby food is absolutely not necessary for baby's development, learning, or growth. With this knowledge in mind, you may be asking: then why is baby food everywhere, and why does everyone think it's so important? That is a story we are eager to share with you.

The Origins of "Baby Food"

New York University professor Amy Bentley has written extensively about the history of baby food in an enlightening book called *Inventing Baby Food: Taste, Health, and the Industrialization of the American Diet.*[17] As she explains in the book, around a hundred years ago, in 1921, a Mrs. Clapp, mother of baby Jack, got sick. Called into baby-feeding duty, Mr. Clapp fed their baby beef broth, vegetables, and cereal, which Jack seemingly liked a lot. Excited by his child's response to his soup, Clapp made a big batch and took it down to the local pharmacy to sell to other parents. This innocuous-sounding anecdote is the basis of today's baby food frenzy, and it launched a cultural attachment to commercial baby food that has become one of the biggest industries today.

A few years after Clapp's Baby Food hit the market, another father began experimenting with strained baby food. This time he wasn't making it for his son but alongside him. Their names were Frank and Dan Gerber.

It was in 1928 that the Gerbers put out a call for an adorable baby to be the face of a campaign selling their food, a marketing idea that launched one of the century's most ubiquitous advertising images. They also enlisted pediatricians to get the word out, despite the lack of research into the products.

The earliest baby foods on the market hit the shelves alongside newly developed infant formulas. Unlike today's formulas, these first formulas lacked nutritional robustness, and formula-fed infants of the day tended not to thrive. The medical community took note and began to recommend iron-rich solid food as early as 4 weeks of age to compensate. As such, many of the earliest baby foods were iron-rich meats like beef, liver, and veal, along with beef and vegetable soups.

Recognizing the market, other companies, including Heinz and Beech-Nut, started producing food for babies as well, and by 1940, an estimated 35 percent of babies in the United States were being fed commercial baby food, and baby food companies were making fifteen million dollars per year.[18] It was around this time that baby food companies began providing doctors with free product to distribute to parents, ensuring that the promises of prepackaged baby food would continue to gain traction.

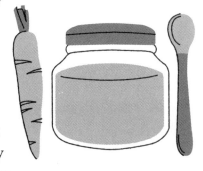

Corporate marketing studies and focus groups soon demonstrated that both baby and mother preferred sweet, fruit-based purees to the iron-rich offerings, and baby food became synonymous with sweetened purees and puddings, catering to baby's innate preference for sweet foods. These fruit purees and custard puddings would soon also be marketed to mothers as a weight-conscious snack, something mothers could eat alongside their baby.

By the 1960s, the average age of starting solids dropped to just 1 month of age, with many babies in the United States being introduced to commercial baby food between 4 and 6 *weeks* of age, dramatically extending the length of time the parent was buying baby food (and that the child was being fed textureless food). It was an excellent time to be in the business of baby food.

What we know now, very clearly, is that this was far too early for babies to be fed solid food of any kind, as the more solids those infants took in, the more it displaced breast milk and formula, which are incredibly important in the first year of life.

Marketing Mom Guilt

The inventors of commercial baby food seemingly had good intentions at the start, wanting to make feeding babies easier. Yet once corporations discovered how profitable it could be, they worked to exploit the most powerful piece of it all: a mother's worry about her child's health.

Early ads were featured prominently in women's magazines. New mothers, with their desire to do things right, were their first target. One notable ad depicts a baby, barely 2 months old, cradled in mother's arms with the caption "What's better than breastfeeding? Breastfeeding and Gerber pears."

For a century, in addition to getting pediatricians to distribute their product, baby food companies have stoked maternal guilt and anxiety in their marketing, from advertisements designed to make new moms question whether their breast milk was enough to whether they were spending too much time in the kitchen.

In another ad by Heinz, beneath an image of a baby on the floor, reaching for mom, the text reads, "Come out of the kitchen, Mother. It's much better for baby!" "Wise mothers today spend more time in the nursery."

Then there were the men's magazine advertisements advising readers that if they were new fathers who "had exchanged their charming wives for tired little mothers," baby food could help.

In the context of the twentieth century, these messages—albeit politically incorrect—were not necessarily wrong: making food for baby did, in fact, keep mothers in the kitchen. Convenience has its place. But what was meant as a campaign to entice parents into buying a product had a number of unintended consequences, including introducing a number of myths into the public consciousness that are still accepted as truths today.

Countering the Myths of Baby Food

One such myth was the idea that baby food was both necessary for infant feeding development and safer than any other food a family might serve. Baby food companies pushed the idea that babies must start with runny, textureless purees and slowly graduate to thicker foods. While this may have been necessary in the 1940s and 1950s when babies were being fed solid food as early as 1 month of age to support nutrition—runny purees are the only texture that a 1-month-old can safely eat—it is no longer considered to be the desired (or necessary) approach. As baby approaches 6 months of age, they have emerging developmental skills that allow them to safely explore and learn to eat a much broader range of textures and food sizes.

"Today we helped Lee start learning how to chew," read one advertisement, depicting a jar of "junior" baby food of pureed beef and egg noodles with "tender particles to encourage chewing" and a silver spoon beside it. "Lee has two front teeth!" the advertisement exclaims, leading the reader to believe that baby is now ready for chewable food. Putting aside the fact that humans don't chew with their front teeth (we chew with our molars, which don't come in until well after baby's first birthday), the assertion that a puree with "tender particles" served from a spoon helped baby learn to chew is just not true. Baby was likely just swallowing unchewed bits of beef and noodles. While mixed-texture purees provide texture exposure, they are ineffective at triggering the reflexes needed to learn to chew. A mostly pureed jar of mush tends to teach baby to suck and swallow their food without chewing. The whole idea of staged baby foods, starting with runny purees and then moving on to gradually thicker and more textured food through stages, may seem logical, but it is inaccurate and not grounded in the science of oral motor development.

We don't believe that baby food companies meant any harm with their staged baby food lines, but regardless of intention, the very existence of those products led generations of parents to assume that it's necessary to buy special foods for every stage in infancy and toddlerhood. And these marketing campaigns argued that if they didn't, mothers would be neglecting their child (and husband). Thankfully, we know better today. And today, the evidence shows us that babies do not need special foods at all, and that in fact, babies flourish when they are invited to share in the family meal.[19]

Doing Away with One-Size-Fits-All

Babies, like adults, come in a wide variety of sizes and shapes, all of which can be perfectly normal. The notion that a preportioned jar of baby food is the perfect amount of food for every baby is problematic. Just as the intake of breast milk or formula can vary widely from infant to infant (and still be the right amount for that given child), the amount of solid food for any given baby will vary widely, depending on baby's genetics, level of activity, growth spurts, and individual nutritional needs. When we look to baby food companies to tell us how much our babies should eat, we are, in essence, looking away from our own baby and their unique needs.

But since the 1970s, concern for and attention to a baby's weight have ballooned, due in large part to the advent of one particular medical tool: growth charts. From the moment one learns they are pregnant, through baby's various checkup appointments, baby is constantly being measured and weighed. Baby's growth has quickly become synonymous with one's success as a parent.

In reality, the range of what is normal for any given baby's size and appetite is wide, as you'll learn in Chapter 15. This is why, at Solid Starts, we don't specify exactly how much solid food a child "should" be eating for any given age. Each baby is unique. What matters most is that you pay attention to your baby—and respond in kind.

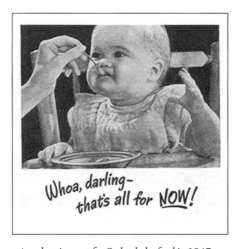

An advertisement for Gerber baby food in 1947.

Even so, for a long time, baby food companies have been exploiting concerns about weight to convince parents and medical professionals alike to embrace their products. Just as baby food advertisements insisted that commercial baby food was necessary, they openly promoted restricting portion sizes—and feeding babies less than they may have wanted, as if a child's hunger was somehow suspicious or wrong instead of the truest indicator that they needed more food in this moment.

"Whoa darling, that's all for now!" read one Gerber ad, warning about the dangers of feeding a hungry baby too much. "When you start your baby on Gerber Cereals, measure out the amount your doctor suggests. Gerber's (ready-to-serve) tastes *so good* even beginners often want more than their share."

Many laugh at these antiquated ads now, but keep in mind that some of them were quite modern in their claims that commercial baby foods were nutritionally superior products. Today, baby food companies continue to lean into this playbook, branding pouches and puffs with terms like "superfood veggies," "smart food for developing brain and body," or "immunity blend," even though these statements are shaky at best when it comes to the science of infant nutrition.

Even the most ample advertising budget can't buy you truth. No matter how much companies spend to market their products, the fact remains that breast milk and infant formula are considered optimal, and should be the main sources of nutrition, for a child's first year of life.[20]

Prepackaged baby foods certainly are easier. But easy doesn't always translate into the desired results. It's time for the medical community to fast-track the translation of research into guidelines that are available and communicated everywhere. All parents need to know that a pouch here and there is one thing, but keeping a child on purees for too long will have consequences.

By 12 to 15 months of age, most children will need to receive the majority of their nutrition from solid foods. Sounds good, but chewing is something babies need many months to learn how to do. Baby can't just flip a switch and turn on those skills on their first birthday. They need time and space for repetitive practice.

Most babies are developmentally ready for food—real food, like you eat—at around 6 to 7 months of age. And by the time you finish reading the next few chapters, you'll be ready, too.

Summary

✓ Recommendations for introducing solid food have changed dramatically over the years.

✓ Today's evidence supports waiting to introduce solids until baby is *developmentally* ready.

✓ The mandatory need for baby food is a myth that has been marketed to the public for a century.

✓ Most babies are ready for real food like we eat around 6 months of age.

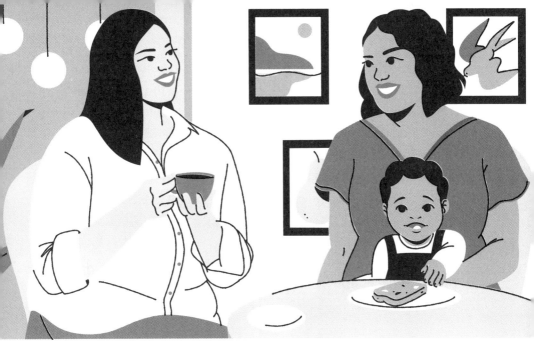

Chapter Three

The Magic of Six Months

William, 6 months old, sits on his mother's lap while she enjoys coffee and a piece of banana bread with her friend at a coffee shop. Before she even realizes what's happening, William has reached out for his mother's breakfast treat and brought it to his mouth, munching away. William is telling his mom, "I'm ready!" and in sharing "adult" foods right now—at 6 months of age—will take advantage of what the research has called a critical window for feeding development.

M ost 6-month-old babies put everything in their mouth: if there's an object within reach, it's going right in their mouth. One of the main ways a baby learns about their environment is through their mouth. And, luckily enough, developmentally they are perfectly set up to sit up and use those arms to get things to their mouth. The 6- to 8-month period is also a time of natural skill building through reflexes, taste, and texture openness. Babies are the most willing they will be to try flavors and textures, and less likely to develop food allergies when exposed to common allergens. That's why we think this time is magical, and why we call it the magic window: it is truly incredible that these opportunities overlap the way that they do while baby is developmentally ready to take advantage of them.

The current research demonstrates that the ideal period for starting solids begins when a baby is about 6 months old and can sit up, can reach for food, and is showing interest. This ideal period closes when baby is around 12 months old.[1,2,3]

During this time, there are three key opportunities that we want to take advantage of:

→ preventing food allergies by introducing allergens early
→ getting baby use to big flavors and textures
→ practicing chewing before key reflexes fade

In addition, during the magic window, breast milk and formula continue to fuel baby's growth, which makes this a beneficial time to explore and practice eating real food without worrying whether baby will consume it.

In this chapter we'll take a close look at why and how to take advantage of this important period of time when baby is most ready and capable of learning to eat.

Preventing Food Allergies

Many food allergies can be prevented, as you'll learn in detail in Chapter 14, by offering foods such as egg, peanut, and cow's milk beginning at around 6 months for most babies and around 4 months for a select few. When common allergens are given early and regularly, many allergies can be staved off in the long run. For example, peanut allergy is 80 percent less likely to develop when babies at high risk of food allergy are introduced to peanut in infancy and it is kept in their diet regularly in early childhood.[4,5] Starting early is key. Waiting too long to introduce peanut can actually *increase* the risk of peanut allergy developing.[6,7] Not every allergy can be prevented, but the evidence for these recommendations is increasingly strong.

Building Baby's Palate

Young babies are incredibly open to new flavors and textures from 6 to 8 months of age. If you want a child who is open to trying new foods, is comfortable with various textures, and is curious about exploring new cuisines, you're going to want to use this magic window of opportunity to get baby accustomed to the wide range of possibility when it comes to food, before their interest in putting things in their mouth fades and toddler neophobia sets in.

Flavors

Just as an infant's brain is optimally open to absorbing and learning new languages if they are exposed to them, infants are highly capable of enjoying a variety of new flavors and textures during this window simply by tasting them over and over again.

This is particularly important because enjoying any new flavor typically requires repeated exposure: the child must be willing to try it over and over again. The more we taste a flavor, the more familiar it becomes, and the more likely our brain will register that flavor as enjoyable. Between 6 and 8 months of age, babies are highly driven to put anything and everything in their mouths, making this window an ideal time to expose baby to a variety of flavors.

Textures

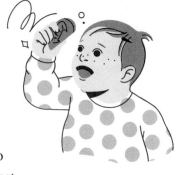

Texture exposure is a little bit more complex. The infant drive to put different textured foods in their mouth pays off in two ways, if we let it. One, babies must learn to tolerate the feel of a new texture in their mouth, and two, they will also need to develop the skills to chew and break down each texture so that it can be swallowed. When a baby is exposed to a particular texture, they get used to how it feels, and they become more likely to accept it and similar textures again in the future. With repeat exposure, they become less likely to refuse foods with a similar texture going forward. With each introduction, they also become more skilled at breaking down that texture. In fact, an infant's chewing patterns are directly impacted by how the texture feels in their mouth: it is in part the texture itself that is influencing their ability to chew it.[8]

The willingness to explore different-textured food and the chewing development that happens in response to this exposure appears to be most powerful from 6 to 8 months of age. In research studies, babies who were exposed to textured and chewable foods during the magic window ate a wider variety of foods as toddlers, were more likely to eat the foods the rest of the family was eating, and were less likely to show signs of selective eating in toddlerhood.[9,10] Children who were exposed to textured and chewable foods *after* 9 months ate statistically fewer fruits and vegetables in toddlerhood and were more selective about what they were willing to eat overall. This has been replicated by multiple studies that have looked at the optimal time to introduce textured and chewable foods to babies in order to prevent later texture aversion, oral motor issues, and selective eating behaviors.[11,12,13,14,15]

Letting Baby Learn to Chew When It's Easiest to Do So

Babies are born with a set of reflexes that will help them learn to chew. These reflexes are why baby will naturally open their mouth, stick out their tongue, bite down, and attempt to chew and move things around the mouth, even from the very first time they are introduced to solids. These reflexes are automatic—baby doesn't need to learn them, they are born with them—but automatic reflexes are not coordinated movements. It will take months of repetitive practice for baby to successfully chew and swallow food. What baby's reflexes do is jump-start the motions needed to learn.

The strong drive to put food in their mouth during the magic window kicks off an important cascade. When food is the right size, shape, and texture, baby's chewing reflexes are triggered. Those reflexes move baby's tongue and jaw automatically in a chewing motion.[16] Take a bite of food. Notice what your tongue immediately does to that food. Mature, coordinated chewing requires the tongue to move food to the side for the gums (and eventually teeth) to grind it. Baby's tongue lateralization reflex does just that and their phasic bite reflex begins to mash the food. As baby explores food that needs to be chewed with their mouth, they're actively building their chewing skills—and purees do not trigger these reflexes.[17,18,19,20] Baby's chewing reflexes are at their strongest in the magic window.

The sooner you start (once baby is showing developmental readiness), the more time baby will have to trigger these reflexes, which helps baby build motor patterns in their brain. As with any activity, the more practice you do, the more skill and coordination you develop. Does this mean a 12-month-old can't learn how to chew if they missed the window? No. Skills can be learned at any age. It's just easier for baby to build chewing skill between 6 and 8 months of age.

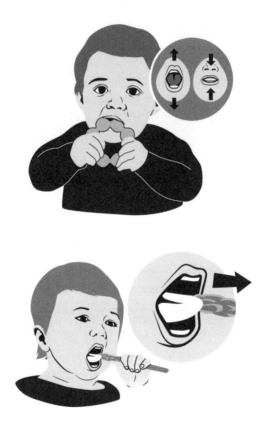

Phasic bite (top) and tongue lateralization are two reflexes that help baby learn to chew.

But what about safety? While we all have innate protections against choking, during the 6- to 8-month window there is also a set of mechanisms that further protect baby's airway and help reduce choking risk. We'll talk about these protective reflexes in subsequent chapters, but for now, know that some of the protective reflexes against choking are at their most powerful and effective from around 6 to 8 months of age and after that, they begin to change, and in some cases disappear. These reflexes, and the mechanisms we discuss below, provide an ideal environment for baby to learn how to chew—and to safely make mistakes. Like wearing a life jacket when learning to swim, the reflexes protect baby from choking while they are learning to eat.

A baby's anatomy between 6 and 8 months of age also provides some protection while baby learns to chew.[21] An infant's face and neck are small, making their mouth and throat structures quite tightly packed together. This means there are fewer open spaces and pockets in their mouth and throat compared to a toddler or older child. This makes food easier to manage and makes swallowing quicker and safer, as there is a very clear and well-defined pathway for food to travel from mouth to stomach. Baby's airway is also positioned higher in their throat, keeping it farther away from where the food passes. Additionally, baby's tongue has a very powerful ability to push things out of the mouth, keeping food far away from the airway. This movement pattern begins to fade as baby learns to move the tongue in more complex ways.

A Nutritional Safety Net

Introducing chewable food between 6 and 8 months of age is also ideal because babies have the nutritional safety net of breast milk or formula to rely upon while they learn and fumble. Just as we would not expect a baby who is learning to walk to be able to walk down the stairs alongside us, we should not expect an infant who is just learning to eat solid food to swallow much at first. At this age, introducing a variety of nourishing foods, particularly iron-rich foods, provides ample opportunity to explore during this phase where baby's nutritional needs start to shift and gradually require iron and other nutrients from solid foods. As baby's self-feeding and chewing skills become stronger, and baby's solid food consumption increases, they will then already have the familiarity with and skill to manage nutritious and iron-rich foods to support their rapid growth, brain development, energy, curiosity, and drive to explore the world around them.

A child who exclusively eats purees off a spoon from 6 to 8 months is not actually practicing a new skill. Spoon-feeding runny purees triggers motor patterns that are very similar to the suck-to-swallow pattern that baby has been using since birth to breast- or bottle-feed. In other words, spoon-feeding purees simply reinforces the skills baby uses to drink breast milk or formula.

Infants who have been fed pouches or spoon-fed purees for long periods of time are more likely to use this liquid-swallowing pattern when trying to eat other foods, which often results in swallowing food whole or excessive gagging once baby is finally introduced to more textured foods.[22] This also delays the practice of new, more complex chewing patterns, as runny purees do not trigger chewing reflexes.

To learn how to chew, baby must be repeatedly offered chewable food.

Missed the Window?

It's okay. Although this is the optimal window for the introduction of solid foods and food allergens, the window for learning never fully closes. Baby's brain can learn the necessary skills after 9 months, as long as you give the right opportunities to practice that skill repetitively. It may be more challenging and take longer to teach a toddler to chew—but, of course, it is not impossible.

If you have not introduced chewable food by 9 months of age and need support in making the transition from spoon-feeding purees to letting baby feed themselves chewable food, jump to Chapter 13. Likewise, if you are late to the game with food allergen introduction, all is not lost. Chapter 14 will help you get back on track.

Anxiety and Why Spoon-Feeding Can Sometimes Help

The research is clear that a parent's anxiety around feeding, and perception of baby's struggles, can be a predictor of later feeding difficulties.[23] It's very challenging to build a trusting relationship with baby during a meal if you are highly anxious.

For nervous parents and caregivers, it can be beneficial to see quick success with spoon-feeding because it can build confidence in baby's ability to make this transition.[24] If jumping right into finger food feels like too much, too fast, spoon-feeding is an option. However, we recommend progressing to self-feeding with the spoon and then finger foods as soon as you feel comfortable. For some families, having the support of an experienced feeding professional can help ease concerns and take this next step forward.

Practice Is Learning

Developing the skills to eat solid foods takes time and is a big challenge for most infants. We cannot expect them to consume much, if anything, for a while. The earlier baby starts chewable food, the more time they have to practice and learn before they have to rely on solid food for nutrition, around 1 year of age.

Taking advantage of the magic window will give baby the consistent practice they need to chew food well and swallow, supporting health and growth in older infancy, toddlerhood, and beyond.

Summary

✓ Between 6 and 8 months is the beginning of a special time of openness, when babies are uniquely ready to learn how to enjoy new flavors and manage textured food.

✓ The 6- to 8-month age window is also a critical time to introduce common allergens such as egg and peanut to help prevent food allergies.

✓ Chewing is most easily learned between 6 to 8 months of age, before key reflexes fade.

✓ Pouches or spoon-feeding purees reinforces oral motor patterns that are similar to sucking, not chewing.

✓ Children who are exposed to a diverse array of chewable food between 6 and 8 months have been shown to eat a wider variety of foods as toddlers.

✓ While it's easiest to build skill in the 6- to 8-month age window, baby can learn later on with the right support.

Part Two

Building Trust

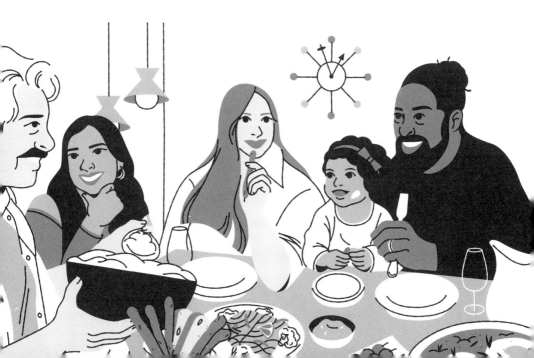

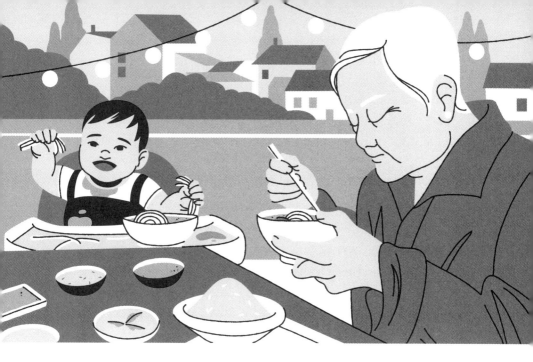

Chapter Four

Building Trust at the Table

Lee, 11 months, and his grandmother are at the table for lunch. They are having noodles in broth—his grandma's favorite. Lee is served the same food, but with less broth since he doesn't know how to use a soup spoon yet. Grandma enjoys her meal, slurping her noodles, and Lee squeals in delight as he explores his, pulling them out of the bowl with his hands, broth dripping all down his arms. When Lee starts to fuss ten minutes later, Grandma asks if he's full. Lee leans out of his high chair in response. Grandma takes that as a sign that he is finished eating and carries him to the sink, where Lee plays with water and washes up.

On its surface, starting solids is about introducing new foods and textures to baby. Considered more deeply, it can be a profound opportunity for relationship building and learning. There's a reason we brought this idea up on the first page of Chapter 1: babies who trust and feel connected to their caregivers are more open and able to learn new skills, hopefully learning to trust their own bodies and internal cues.[1] While you are learning to trust baby at the table, baby is learning to trust you—and to trust themself.

For families, this is a chance to welcome baby into the joyful, fun, exciting world of food and flavor and cultural practices, and to show them how much you believe in them. It can also be a time of anxiety for many parents and caregivers. Letting baby take a bite of food when all they have ever known is breast milk or formula can feel scary—especially if you have never seen this in action before. You may be thinking, "Is this safe?" or "Can baby handle this?" Baby will very likely have questions of their own: "What is this?" "What happens if I put it in my mouth?" You will need to look to one another for answers and reassurance, because working together is essential.

Earning Baby's Trust

We have worked with thousands of families over the years who are trying to mend broken trust at the table, which can happen when parents exert too much control. One of the quickest ways to scramble baby's beautiful and balanced inherent system of curiosity, exploration, and hunger and fullness is by trying to insert too much control— control over whether baby eats at any given meal and how much they eat, control

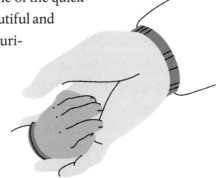

of the mess, and control over the activity each time baby fumbles or struggles even a small amount.

Overriding baby's desire to learn and explore can be quite challenging to undo. It may lead to months and sometimes years of work trying to return to a place of internal motivation and joy at mealtimes. That's why we will always stress the importance of giving baby space to learn even when it gets messy and takes more time. And it's why we focus on learning how to interpret and respect baby's natural cues of engagement and disengagement, and eventually, hunger and fullness.

We earn baby's trust at the table in a few ways. We earn it by showing our trust in them, by giving baby space to explore food without disrupting them, by respecting baby's communications, and by trusting their body's ability to learn new skills and to regulate hunger. We also earn their trust by being as consistent as possible in our responses, and by showing joy in their efforts. When baby trusts you, they are most open to learning from you, naturally mimicking your behaviors and actions, and they feel safe to try, fail, and try again.

Give Baby Space for Repetitive Practice

Infants move the equivalent distance of seven football fields every hour as they practice the movements needed to walk.[2] They try out different patterns, they fall, and then they try again, across varied environments and surfaces. They crawl on grass, hardwood, carpet, and concrete, and learn to change their movement patterns to make each environment work. They problem solve, change directions, and keep going. Researchers conclude that as infants are learning to walk, they are learning to learn—to anticipate and adapt to any environment.[3]

Learning to eat is strikingly similar. The transition to solid food is all about learning to chew but also about learning to problem solve and to manage change, disappointment, and struggle, while developing resilience and confidence in a new task. When babies encounter new textures and new environments, they are learning to adapt their skills to the unfamiliar, to anticipate, and to change. Most infants are born with the ability to take in liquids (sucking and swallowing are automatic reflexes), but chewing and eating safely are entirely new skills that take considerable precision and coordination. Chewing is built on innate reflexes, too, but those reflexes need to be stimulated over and over again, with a wide variety of foods that react differently in the mouth. Repetitive yet varied practice is necessary to build these skills and to learn to learn. Their job is to practice. Yours is to trust that all this practice is leading baby in the right direction.

Baby has likely already demonstrated that they can learn an incredible amount in a very short period of time. Baby has learned to roll, to hold their head upright, and to use their arms purposefully—to grab hold of items, pass things back and forth between their hands, and bring them to their mouth. These are wildly complex skills and baby likely figured this all out quite naturally. If baby is developing as expected so far and is healthy, they can likely start learning to eat solids, too, if you give them the chance. Not immediately, of course, but gradually over the next few months they will explore and lay a strong foundation of skills for eating.

Watching for Communication About Hunger and Fullness

Humans are born with an inherent drive to seek out food. When a hungry baby has the opportunity to eat, most are very motivated to do so. Babies are also born with a drive to stop eating when the belly feels full. Trusting that nearly all children have a strong internal motivation to eat when they are hungry and stop when they are full is central to teaching baby to trust themself and their inner cues. This idea—that children have a powerful inherent motivation to eat when they are hungry and stop when they feel full—is an important concept that we'll come back to frequently throughout this book.

As important as this is, baby has time to get there. Right at first, baby doesn't even know that food at the table is food at all. They do not know that a spoonful of puree or a piece of food can be eaten and will help fill their belly. In fact, it's not hunger that prompts baby to reach out and try to eat something you serve right at first.

Baby is motivated to explore food in the same way they are motivated to explore a toy: they want to put it in their mouth to figure out what it is and how it works. Eventually, baby understands that these aren't toys at all, but rather a special new category of object that offers a point of connection with their caregivers, can be eaten, is delicious, and can help baby feel full. This lightbulb moment usually happens closer to 9 to 12 months for most babies, though some figure it out earlier and others a bit later.

Baby's behavior is how they communicate. These behaviors tell you when they are interested in exploring a food and when they are not, and after a while this will transition to communicating that they are hungry and full. Pay attention to them. A baby's communication can be both overt and subtle. Baby may turn their head away as an indication that they need a break, or they may begin screaming as a more overt "I'm done" cue. Interpreting their communication and responding accordingly is an essential part of building trust between you and baby. Baby needs to know that you are listening to them and you care about what they have to say.

Trusting Baby Starts with Trusting Yourself

If trusting baby to know how much food their own body needs feels scary to you, you are not alone. We've been told overtly and subconsciously for decades that babies are not to be trusted; they need constant weighing and measuring, plus special baby foods made just for them. The assumptions and feelings you have around feeding baby are interwoven with history, culture, and your own food journey as a child.

Trusting baby at the table starts with trusting yourself. If you are a parent, you know your baby better than anyone and you know baby's cues, behaviors, and temperament. You know what's typical for baby and what is not. If you are a caregiver or a medical professional who works with infants, you know the difference between a calm, happy baby and a very fussy, unhappy one. Trust these signs to guide you when it comes to feeding baby. There will be small challenges and moments when you think something is off. We will walk you through many common issues that arise with baby later in this book. Trust that you have the skills to modify and adapt as needed to help baby be successful at the table. And trust that you will know in your gut when to seek more support if needed.

Many parents make it to adulthood with strained relationships with food and their bodies. Trusting baby to feed themself and to eat the amount they need can be even more challenging if you have experienced disordered eating. You may not be sure how to trust baby because you may not trust yourself. Take a moment to reflect on and acknowledge any food rules you may have. Gently challenge yourself to see that all food has a place on the table and that balance is key. Complex and challenging feelings around the body, while painful, are common. Extend yourself grace and self-compassion as you reflect on the type of body image environment you'd like to live in, for yourself and for baby.

Research tells us that a parent's or caregiver's relationship with food influences how they feed their child and that children as young as 3 years of age have expressed negative feelings about their bodies.[4,5,6,7] The negative comments made about a child's body have lasting emotional impact.[8,9]

This time in life, the postpartum period, is one in which neuroplasticity—the brain's ability to grow and change—is quite high for parents.[10] That makes right now an excellent time to reflect on beliefs you may have been carrying around, and challenge negative feelings you may have about food. Baby's start with solid food is also a valuable opportunity for you to acknowledge any fractured relationship you may have with food and possibly create change that the whole family can benefit from.

The Long-Game Benefits of Building Trust

Trust and a positive relationship at the table will gradually permeate all aspects of life for baby.[11] The research on eating together—and the benefits it bestows on children of all ages—is robust.[12] These mealtimes do not need to be complicated in order to make a big impact.

Consider this exciting fact: all humans have what are called mirror neurons, which are brain cells that light up as powerfully when we see someone else do something as when we do it ourselves.[13,14] Eating with baby cues up the mirror neurons, prompting them to imitate you. This imitation helps them learn how to eat. It also gives them a chance to learn social and emotional skills, as modeled by you. Every supportive word you give and every time you model patience, respect, problem solving, and flexibility builds on the last, teaching baby how to move through the world with these skills.

Many parents and caregivers feel like baby's schedule prohibits eating together, and it can be tricky to pull off. There are small steps you can take even in the early months of starting solids when baby's eating and sleep schedule may differ from your own. Getting into the habit of eating together now keeps the long game in mind. Eating together might look like:

→ sitting next to baby and eating while they eat
→ taking a taste of their yogurt with your own spoon or finger
→ sharing a snack on the floor

For babies, mealtime is a chance to develop the crucial habits, skills, and beliefs that will impact how they feel about eating and how they move through the world in the years that follow: joyful mealtimes together help support positive mental health outcomes for your child even through their teenage years.[15]

Let Them Fumble

For babies, learning to eat is complex work, with many skills to be honed. It's going to take a lot of time for baby to successfully eat a bite of food, let alone a full meal. This is okay and expected. Trust that the skills baby is learning at every meal build on the last.

It can be challenging to know how much they are swallowing at first. Thankfully, breast milk and formula are still providing most of baby's nutrition, and even small amounts of food allergens provide protective benefits. Let this free you from feeling worried or pressured to calculate how much they're getting from those early solid meals. Aim to focus on learning and building skill, not intake.

Trust that baby is fully capable of figuring this out. Yes, they will make mistakes. Picking the food up, losing grip, dropping it, eventually getting it to their mouth, munching, spitting, storing food in their cheeks—these are not a by-product of the process but an essential part of it. This is known as *instinctive fumbling,* and it is how babies learn. All these fumbles eventually get them to the goal—eating the foods you and your family enjoy. So when you see baby struggling, remember that this is what learning looks like. Not like a lightbulb moment, but like a series of missteps. They learn through trial and error, not by getting it right the first, second, or even fifth time. They learn through the mistakes, the fumbling, how to get back up and do it again, and better.

When you want to step in, hang back for a moment; even if it gets a little uncomfortable for you, you can take comfort in knowing that baby's reflexes and physiology help get them started and offer protection from harm, giving baby the space they need to fumble through in order to learn the rest.

Letting babies learn to chew and develop their skills in infancy teaches them that they can accomplish what they set out to do, even when it is challenging. Every meal is an opportunity to support them at the table, assuring them that you are their go-to for guidance in all areas of life. Parents, remember, you are baby's North Star. They can only do all of this hard work because of your guidance—a supportive, connected caregiver in whom they have trust.

Summary

✓ Let trust be a guiding principle. Trust in baby's ability to sense when they are hungry and when they are full and in your ability to support their developing self-awareness.

✓ Exerting too much control at meals, such as refusing to let baby hold their utensil or insisting on them taking another bite, can interrupt baby's natural system of curiosity and desire to learn.

✓ Don't worry about how much food baby is swallowing at the start. Babies have the nutritional safety net of breast milk or formula to rely upon while they learn.

✓ Baby is watching you to learn how to eat—and to learn how to feel about food. If you have a strained relationship with food, you are not alone. Now is a great time to hold compassion for yourself as you work through this, as you simultaneously learn alongside baby.

✓ Let baby fumble. We all learn when we make mistakes.

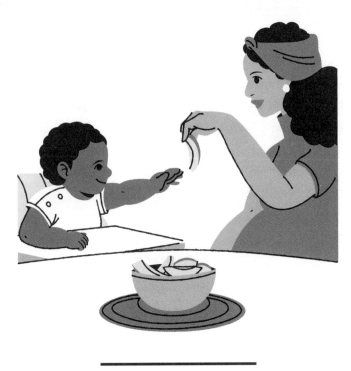

Chapter Five

Responsive Feeding

Essie, 6 months old, is a small baby according to her pediatrician. She struggled with breastfeeding and ultimately transitioned to full bottle-feeding by 2 months old, but she continued to be slow to gain weight. She is starting solids today and her parents, worried about weight gain, attempt to spoon-feed her at first. Essie is sitting well in her high chair, and when her mom brings the spoon toward her she immediately makes eye contact, smiles, and reaches for the spoon, trying to grab it. This interest delights and surprises her parents, who try to help her balance the spoon but within a few bites realize that Essie wants to be in control. They continue to help her load the spoon whenever she sets it down, and once Essie loses interest in the activity (when she stops reaching out for the spoon and instead starts looking around the room and fussing), they end the meal. Twenty minutes later, they offer Essie a bottle.

R esponsive feeding is trust in action. If you know what responsive feeding is, you're already a step ahead of the game. If not, by the end of this chapter, you'll be well-versed in what it is, why it's important, and how you can use it to benefit baby's relationship with food.

At its core, responsive feeding is about connecting with baby instead of trying to control them, about learning how to communicate and understand their signals so that you and baby can cultivate a partnership, each with your own set of responsibilities when it comes to eating. As we will explain, it's your role to provide the food. Baby's job is to determine if they want to eat, and how much, as you support along the way.

Connection Is a Biological Need

It was once believed that the significance of the infant-caregiver relationship was founded primarily in the infant's need to be fed. That is not actually the case. In fact, connection to a caregiver is a biological need all its own that is separate from hunger and the need for food. But while these drives for hunger and connection are separate, they intersect in countless important ways.

Responsive feeding emerged from the research on attachment theory and responsive parenting. Per attachment theory, humans have a deep need to connect and form a close emotional bond with a caregiver, and if their caregiver is appropriately responsive, an infant will develop this bond early in life.[1,2] Attachment was once considered fringe, but the evidence base has mounted to demonstrate its critical impact, and we now know that attachment supports growth, independence, emotional development, and mental health. Responsive parenting, which grew in popularity in response to the hands-off, discipline-heavy parenting practices of the first half of the twentieth century, is a style of parenting that is highly empathetic and leads with connection while holding appropriate boundaries. Caregivers place themselves in the role of teacher—not boss or friend—and emphasize learning over compliance and obedience.

In 2000, researchers coined the term "responsive feeding," a principle in which the infant communicates hunger or fullness, and the caregiver responds to those cues.[3] Responsive feeding holds similar tenants to responsive parenting—that feeding a child should be approached with a mix of connection, communication, and boundaries.

Here's what this means for you: in the beginning, baby will express to you in a variety of ways that they are hungry, and you will respond by offering the breast or a bottle. When you do this, baby learns that their communication has power, they can voice their needs, their needs matter, and their needs will be met. In turn, our ability to understand baby grows along with our connection. Caregivers trust that baby knows what they need or want, and baby trusts that their caregiver will listen. This reciprocity is crucial for nursing or bottle-feeding, and the goal is to continue to build on this patterning when starting solid foods.

A Note on Attachment Theory

Early research on attachment theory lacked cultural inclusion and sensitivity, and the depth and breadth of the research is expanding.[4,5] It's worthwhile to acknowledge that attachment varies across cultures and can come in many healthy shapes and forms.

You Provide, the Child Decides

One of the most effective ways to put responsive feeding into action is something called the "division of responsibility." This practice helps clarify what the parent is in charge of and what we should leave up to baby.[6] The simplest version of this is "you provide, child decides." As the caregiver, you control the *what, where, and when*—things like the menu, the time of the meal, and where you eat, as well as your attitude when you show up to the feeding experience. Baby decides what to eat and how much. This can be used as a flexible structure and exceptions may be needed, but it can help you focus on your role and the elements of a meal within your control.

To be responsive, parents and caregivers must pay attention to baby. All of baby's behaviors—things like turning their head, stiffening their body, smiling, pushing you or an object away, reaching out, closing eyes, holding on, letting go, babbling, laughing—are communicating something. Yes, babies have all sorts of random movements and behaviors, but they are remarkably communicative and purposeful most of the time. Look for the signs of communication. Use your own experiences and knowledge to try to interpret what they mean.

Developmental specialists call these signs "cues of engagement or disengagement" and often break them down into "approach" signs and "avoid" signs, meaning signs that baby wants to engage and is ready to learn versus signs that baby is becoming upset, needs a break, or is done.

Common approach signs:

Smiling	Maintaining a calm demeanor
Laughing	Babbling
Making eye contact	Reaching out or leaning in

Common avoid signs:

Closing eyes

Looking away/turning head

Hiccuping

Sneezing repeatedly

Stiffening the body

Arching away

Pushing an object away

Fussing or crying

Yawning

When you see signs of approach, baby is telling you they are ready for and interested in learning. They are saying "teach me," but, because babies learn best by doing, they are also saying "let me try." At the table, look for when baby reaches out for the food, leans toward it, opens their mouth, and shows eagerness to do what you are doing.

Example of Responsive Feeding in Action

Let's return to Essie's story and her family. Essie's parents were worried about her intake and growth. They were eager to learn new patterns and behaviors but were carrying with them fear about her weight gain. Let's walk through how they followed responsive feeding practices while spoon-feeding her:

- ☐ They waited for her to be interested in the feeding experience (developmentally and cognitively).
- ☐ They closely watched her behavior and responded appropriately by letting her grasp the spoon when she reached out. (This is called "responsive spoon-feeding.")
- ☐ They let her fumble through getting the spoon to her mouth but helped with reloading it each time.
- ☐ They shared their delight and excitement in her exploration— the focus was on her learning, not the volume consumed.
- ☐ They ended the meal when Essie communicated with her actions that she was losing interest.

Responsive Spoon-Feeding

When feeding a baby via spoon, it's important to follow responsive spoon-feeding practices. Responsive spoon-feeding is where a caregiver provides the spoon and waits for the baby to reach for the spoon (or lean in and open their mouth to accept the food). Responsive spoon-feeding avoids things like counting how many bites baby accepts or trying to "trick them" into eating any specific amount. There is no "right" amount of food for a baby to eat—the task at hand is for baby to explore the food texture and flavor and learn about it.

If you are feeling anxious, it's okay to move more slowly through baby's solid food journey. You can provide opportunities for responsive spoon-feeding—but after a while, you'll likely see them reach for the spoon, try to bring it to their own mouth, and take control. In fact, nearly all babies are driven to do so around 6 to 7 months of age.

It's been one month since Essie started solids, and she often refuses to reach for the spoon. Her parents tried pulling out a new puree when this happened, which usually got Essie interested again. But now Essie is consistently turning her head and avoiding the spoon, no matter how many new food choices her parents try. She will happily sit at the table and still loves to watch her siblings eat, but she is no longer interested in the foods offered to her. Her parents wonder if she isn't hungry enough or if something else is wrong.

In this situation, Essie's family made an educated guess about what they thought she was communicating. What they missed was her interest in what the family was eating and how they were eating it. Essie was not communicating that she needed different flavors; remember, most 6-month-olds are naturally driven to explore most flavors. What she was communicating was a readiness for more control: to eat with her own hands.

> Essie's parents do away with the spoon for a while and move on to offering her finger foods. As they give her the chance to explore what the rest of the family is eating and the opportunity to eat with her own hands, Essie's interest quickly picks back up. A few weeks into this, however, Essie's parents hit a bump in the road. Essie was happily exploring solid foods but now stops as soon as she becomes frustrated. If she can't quite keep her grip on a slippery item or if she bites off a piece of food, she becomes upset and so her parents end the meal. Her parents aren't sure what to do and they feel the meals aren't going well. They worry she is not eating enough.

A 6- to 12-month-old baby is highly capable of learning to eat food, but learning is challenging, and baby may become frustrated as they struggle to figure it out. But remember, this struggle is extraordinarily beneficial. When baby communicates things like frustration, upset, or confusion, it's natural as a parent to want to fix it, to make the upset go away. Quite often, though, baby does not actually need this. Baby needs a small amount of support—what we call scaffolding—to help them along the way and allow them to complete the task on their own.[7,8]

Creating Scaffolding for Learning

Scaffolding is a process where a parent or caregiver teaches by show-ing, then provides just enough support to help a child do it on their own. Scaffolding helps a child learn something that is just beyond their current capabilities. The caregiver provides the "just right chal-lenge," necessitating some persistence and effort, but the activity is achievable enough to keep baby motivated to try.[9] When you provide scaffolding for baby, try to think about giving the *least* amount of sup-port necessary to enable them to continue to work independently.[10]

In Essie's case, she struggled with some of the activity of feeding herself and when this happened, her parents took this as a sign the meal should end. Some parents may also jump to feeding the child or offering different foods. However, there is a lot to learn from this struggle. Essie was perfectly capable of figuring out feeding herself on her own—with a bit more time and effort and some soothing encour-agement from her parents. Of course, if she was really struggling or if their attempts at scaffolding only led to more frustration, ending the meal is a good way to go.

But there are a few ways Essie's parents could scaffold the task to see if she could keep going and build upon the skills she already had. They could try picking the food up and handing it over to allow her to grab it more successfully. They could try cutting notches in the food so she could get a better grip. And if Essie couldn't calm herself, they could try holding her on their lap for the meal, giving her some extra connection while she worked hard at learning to eat. All these small steps allow Essie to keep learning how to eat solids.

Often there are many small ways we can provide an element of support without jumping in and taking over. Sometimes all baby needs is a smile or a soothing voice to help them feel seen and calm enough to keep trying. Do not underestimate the power of your pres-ence as a loving caregiver to soothe baby and help them do some-thing challenging. Sometimes they may need you to pick them up and hold them for a few minutes to help them regulate. They may also need a little bit of playful interaction to engage with or continue engaging with the food. All these small steps can have a big impact on baby's ability to figure out how to self-feed, chew, and eat alongside you. This is the dance of connection and responsiveness that happens at each meal.

Trust in Action

In essence, responsive feeding requires the parent and caregivers to simultaneously trust baby and let go, while observing baby closely for signs of communication, and respond. It's normal to be unsure about what baby is communicating. Make your best guess. Responsiveness takes trial and error, and you may misinterpret baby's needs or wants at first, but you'll learn from each other with time and become better and better at translating baby's cues.

Responsive feeding is looking for baby to show you that they're ready, and for parents and caregivers to show that they trust baby enough to let go of control and allow baby to lead. These moments are essential to raising happy eaters, and they will come around frequently at the table and beyond. In fact, they will start coming more and more frequently with every month that passes. While it may be challenging to let go—perhaps because of the mess, a fear of choking, or worry that baby will not eat enough—letting go and getting out of the way allows baby to continue to grow, learn, and be heard.

Stopping baby from grabbing a utensil or keeping them from taking the lead communicates "I don't trust that you can do this" and "I can do it better." Over time, this can lead to frequent food refusal on baby's part (or a battle of wills with a very strong-willed baby who disagrees with you) and, in many cases, a child giving up. Instead, you can be baby's first cheerleader. As they explore food, baby will make mistakes and have to deal with frustrations. They will use problem-solving skills. Your loving and supportive presence, scaffolding, and active modeling give baby the sense of security they need to manage this—and so much more.

Summary

✓ Responsive feeding is trust in action: the caregiver pays attention to baby's nonverbal communication and responds in kind.

✓ Signs that baby wants to engage and learn include leaning in, smiling, eye contact, babbling, and reaching. This is an optimal time to practice the new skills of eating solids.

✓ Signs that baby needs a break or is done can include looking away, yawning, sneezing repeatedly, stiffening, arching back, crying, or pushing things away.

✓ Your role is to provide the food. Baby's job is to determine how much they want to eat.

✓ Scaffolding helps baby build skill. You show baby how and create a supportive environment so that baby can succeed. Then you step back and give them the space to try it out.

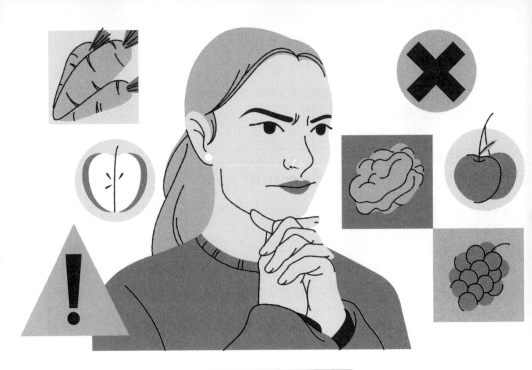

Chapter Six

Overcoming the Fear of Choking

As a first-time mom, I am really anxious about starting solids. My 9-month-old, Theo, has been eating purees for 3 months now and today I offered him a piece of avocado and he immediately bit off a piece. My heart just about stopped but then he spit it out and I quickly took it all away. I want to try again but even thinking about it sends me through the roof thinking he's going to choke on his food.

—Danielle

TRIGGER WARNING: This chapter discusses infant death as we discuss how rare it is for a baby to die from choking.

The possibility of a baby choking is terrifying. It is that fear that leads many parents to opt for the comfort of baby food when they begin to offer solids. By the time you finish this chapter, you'll understand that choking is *not* a common cause of death in babies or young children.[1] You will also understand why delaying the introduction of chewable food past 9 months of age may actually *increase* the risk of choking once chewable food is introduced.[2,3,4,5]

Unraveling Myths About Self-Feeding

Parents and medical professionals alike are often surprised to learn that historical recommendations for feeding babies are lacking in research and evidence. Questions like "What is the most effective way to help a baby learn to chew?" and "What is the safest way to introduce a baby to solids?" were not explored until recently. When baby food companies began making claims about infant feeding development and safety in the 1920s and 1930s, these claims were accepted as facts, despite the lack of unbiased research to support them.[6]

As a result, many families resorted to what their own parents did before them. Like many aspects of parenting, a rationale for "doing it the way it was always done" developed over the years and carried forward into future generations. A similar pattern held true for medical professionals. When it comes to feeding infants, three particularly pervasive myths have been passed down from generation to generation:

1 **Myth 1:** Babies and children are more likely to die from choking than adults.

2 **Myth 2:** Babies can't have food that needs to be chewed until they have teeth.

3 **Myth 3:** Spoon-feeding baby food is safer than letting baby feed themself chewable food.

These myths—however logical seeming—are not true. This matters because each of these myths, if taken as truths, can cause problems in infant feeding in both the short and long term. Let's break down these myths to help debunk them and ease your mind.

Myth #1
Babies are more likely to die from choking than adults.

Contrary to popular belief, choking is *not* a common cause of death in babies and children.[7] Approximately 1 out of every 100,000 infants will die from choking on an object or food each year. Compared to young children (ages 1 through 4), children (ages 5 through 17), and adults, the data is nearly the same. After age 50, the rate of death from choking increases, and that risk continues to increase with age. By the time an adult reaches age 80 through 84, the rate of death jumps to about 10 out of every 100,000 adults each year.

But even for an elderly adult, the risk is low; choking is not a major cause of death. Not in infancy, childhood, or adulthood. Choking accounts for *less than* 1 percent of deaths in babies and children under age 4.[8] And when we isolate choking incidents for those just involving food (as opposed to objects such as coins or small toys), the percentage is reduced even more to a small fraction of a percent. Choking is by no means a common or frequent cause of death or serious injury.

Myth #2
Babies are not ready for chewable food until they have teeth.

It is a misconception that babies need teeth to eat. In fact, the teeth that humans use to chew (molars) typically don't come in until after a baby's first birthday, usually between 13 and 19 months of age.[9] Babies can safely munch and grind age-appropriate food with their gums.

While it's logical to assume that babies need teeth to eat any solid food at all, the fallacy has been reinforced by messaging in advertisements for baby food. For clarity, babies don't chew with their front teeth. The front teeth are used for biting and tearing, which baby cannot do when lumpy baby food is served on a spoon. In fact, that lumpy baby food is most likely to be sucked-to-swallowed or mashed against the palate with the tongue because the pieces in it are not big enough to stimulate the body's chewing reflexes. Baby food has been marketed as the "training wheels" of learning to chew, when in fact the majority of these products just delay the learning process.

Myth #3

Spoon-feeding baby food is safer than letting baby feed themself chewable food.

Along with the myth perpetuated by baby food companies that babies need teeth to eat is the myth that textureless baby food is safer than letting baby feed themself chewable food. The research tells us this simply isn't true: a two-year randomized controlled trial conducted in New Zealand demonstrated that babies who were permitted to start solids by feeding themselves appropriate foods did *not* choke more frequently compared to their spoon-fed peers at any age.[10]

We also know from physiology research that when an individual feeds themself, the risk of choking generally *decreases*.[11,12,13] There is immense brain activation that occurs well before the food ever makes its way into the mouth. Reaching out, touching the food, and picking up the food gives the brain vital sensory information about how the food will feel and likely move within the mouth, which increases attention, readiness to chew, and the ability to manage that food.

As a person chooses to bring the food toward their lips, the brain kicks in to start the chewing process, causing the mouth to open and the tongue to move, prepping the swallow reflex to activate safely and efficiently.[14] All of these work together to help safely manage and swallow food. The research about the importance of self-feeding began in nursing homes, though this has been replicated in pediatrics. Studies of geriatric patients show that when older adults are fed by another person, choking is more likely to occur. Adults who are allowed to feed themselves are more engaged in the eating process and are at lower risk of choking.[15,16,17]

While there is no harm in spending a week or so spoon-feeding purees to a baby who is just getting started with solids, do not forget that spoon-feeding purees is not an effective way to teach baby to chew. And the research on critical windows of oral motor development tells us that waiting for a baby to grow older or sprout more teeth before introducing chewable food does not decrease the risk of choking—it may increase it. As professionals who specialize in the neurobiology of swallowing and the physiology of choking, we're not worried about the 6-month-old munching on a large piece of food; we're worried about the 12-month-old toddler who's never had any practice with chewable food. Why? Because that toddler is more mobile and more likely to be offered—at daycare, school, or parties—high-risk foods marketed for kids such as gummy fruit snacks and baby carrots.

Of equal importance is the fact that the anatomy of an infant airway, which is protective against choking, begins to change in toddlerhood.[18] And some of the protective reflexes against choking in the 12-month-old toddler are just not as easily triggered as they are in an infant. In other words, it's likely harder for a baby to choke than it is for a toddler to choke on the same food. Delaying the introduction of chewable foods and spoon-feeding baby for an extended period of time can slow down the practice of important chewing skills during a period of time when baby's protective reflexes against choking are in high gear.

Understanding the Data Around Choking

The death of any infant or child is heart-wrenching. But looking at the data on choking can give parents much-needed perspective on this fear, as well as help reframe the conversation for medical professionals and policy makers who may make health recommendations that could prevent future deaths. So here, we'll take a look at what the evidence shows us, specifically, a five- and ten-year collection of mortality data from the U.S. Centers for Disease Control and Prevention (CDC). (The National Center for Health Statistics at the CDC tracks causes of death for children and adults in America based on death certificates.) Choking deaths due to food or objects account for less than 1 percent or about twenty deaths per year among 4- to 11-month-old infants in the United States, a number that pales in comparison to the number of infants who die from sudden infant death syndrome (SIDS), unsafe sleep, homicide, and more (page 58).

Choking on food or another object accounts for 1.6 percent of total toddler deaths each year in the United States. In addition to those listed in the graph on page 59, more common causes of death than choking include drowning, homicide, cancer, and pedestrian accidents.

As we mentioned earlier, when you look further into the data on choking, an interesting picture emerges. When we isolate choking incidents in infants involving food (as opposed to objects such as coins or small toys), the percentage lowers significantly to just 0.2 percent. That means more babies die each year from choking on objects (like a toy part) versus food, whereas among toddlers under age 4 there are more deaths from choking on food versus objects. There is no way to know the full story behind each death in the CDC data, but this breakdown of infant and toddler choking deaths is quite fascinating. The risk of death from choking on food does not improve between infancy and toddlerhood.

Top 5 Causes of Infant Death Among 4- through 11-month-olds in the United States, 2017–2021		
Cause of infant death	Average number of deaths per year in the U.S.	Percentage of total infant deaths
Congenital malformations and chromosomal abnormalities	504.6	16.9%
Sudden Infant Death Syndrome (SIDS)	457.6	15.3%
Suffocation or strangulation due to unsafe sleep conditions	318.0	10.7%
Diseases of the heart and circulatory system	158.0	5.3%
Assault/homicide	127.8	4.3%
Choking on a food or an object	20.2	0.68%
Choking on an object	13.2	0.44%
Choking on food	7	0.22%

Top 5 Causes of Death in Infants (4 months through 11 months), as well as choking-related deaths in the United States between 2017 and 2021. "Choking on food or objects" refers to deaths due to inhalation and ingestion of food or other objects causing obstruction of respiratory tract.

Source: Centers for Disease Control and Prevention, National Center for Health Statistics. National Vital Statistics System, Linked Birth / Infant Deaths on CDC WONDER Online Database. Data are from the Linked Birth / Infant Deaths Records 2017–2021, as compiled from data provided by the 57 vital statistics jurisdictions through the Vital Statistics Cooperative Program. Accessed at http://wonder.cdc.gov/lbd-current-expanded.html on Jan 1, 2024.

You may be wondering if we can determine the feeding history (self-fed or spoon-fed) of infants and toddlers who have died from choking, but unfortunately this data does not exist. What we do know is that there has not been an increase in year-to-year deaths due to

Top 5 Causes of Toddler Death Among 1- through 3-year-olds in the United States, 2011–2020 data		
Cause of toddler death	Average number of deaths per year in the U.S.	Percentage of total foddler deaths
Congenital malformations and chromosomal abnormalities	383.4	11.6%
Drowning	354.6	10.7%
Assault/homicide	296.3	9.0%
Cancer	245.5	7.4%
Motor vehicle accident	162.3	4.9%
Choking on a food or an object	54.4	1.64%
Choking on an object	22.5	0.68%
Choking on food	31.9	0.96%

Top 5 Causes of Death in Toddlers (12 months through 3 years), as well as choking-related deaths in the United States between 2011 and 2020. "Choking on food or objects" refers to deaths due to inhalation and ingestion of food or other objects causing obstruction of respiratory tract.

Source: Centers for Disease Control and Prevention, National Center for Health Statistics. National Vital Statistics System, Mortality 1999–2020 on CDC WONDER Online Database, released in 2021. Data are from the Multiple Cause of Death Files, 1999–2020, as compiled from data provided by the 57 vital statistics jurisdictions through the Vital Statistics Cooperative Program. Accessed at http://wonder.cdc.gov/ucd-icd10.html on Jan 2, 2024.

infants choking on food as the concept of self-feeding solids has spread across the United States, and research has not found any increase in choking frequency between infants who self-fed solids compared to their spoon-fed peers.[19] It is important to also keep in mind that when it comes to assessing choking risk, there are several factors to be considered outside of the shape and characteristic of a particular food, which we will discuss later on in this chapter.

Analyzing the mortality data from the CDC, we know that each year, about 2,990 infants 4 through 11 months of age and about 3,310 toddlers age 1 through 3 years die. On average, 7 infant choking deaths (4 through 11 months of age) and 32 toddler choking deaths (age 1 through 3 years) are caused by food each year. To help put things in perspective, each year there are on average 458 infant deaths (4 through 11 months of age) due to SIDS and an average of 355 toddler deaths (age 1 through 3 years) related to drowning (see pages 58 and 59).

Despite the data that shows that death or serious injury by choking is not a top risk for babies and toddlers, media and advertising often underscore the dangers of choking. From advertisements for baby food to anti-choking suction devices to well-meaning media outlets misinterpreting the data, parents are inundated with messaging that stokes fear. For example, we commonly see "One child dies every five days from choking," which sounds very frequent. But in this instance, "child" is defined as any person under the age of 18, and when you do the math, it comes out to be about 73 per year—which aligns with the data outlined previously. This headline is made to make parents feel that death by choking is very common.

We have also observed that media outlets incorrectly cite choking as a "leading cause of death of young children," which we think stems from how the CDC categorizes fatality data. When someone uses the National Center for Health Statistics Mortality Data on the CDC WONDER database and runs a report for "15 Leading Causes of Death," the category "Accidents (unintentional injuries)" results as one of the top five causes of death for both infants and toddlers. While choking is one small part of the overall category of Accidents, choking is *not* a leading cause of death and never has been—for any age. In short, our fear of choking is out of proportion with the statistical likelihood.

When Choking Isn't Choking

Another reason choking is so prominent in the discourse around child safety is the fact that many other incidents get labeled as "choking," when in fact the child is not choking at all. Gagging, coughing, and even infant reflux symptoms (while eating) are often misinterpreted as choking because they have vaguely similar or even overlapping symptoms to choking, which can confuse people. What's more, the term "choking" is often used by parents and medical professionals alike as a shorthand for any sort of difficulty eating or swallowing, even when they know that what happened was not actually a life-threatening emergency. It's not uncommon to hear a parent say, "Baby choked a little," when the baby is clearly breathing and comfortable but coughed a few times while eating. True choking is a life-threatening emergency, and it cannot be easily resolved without help. Choking requires emergency intervention in the form of back blows or chest/abdominal thrusts to use air pressure in the lungs to forcefully expel the item.

We hear from hundreds of parents every day in emails and direct messages, and we pay very close attention to the occasional messages that mention choking. Some parents are anxious. Some are terrified. Some want to tell us about the time their child choked and want guidance and reassurance on how to move forward. Here's the reassurance we offer to these parents and to you: very few of the messages we get from parents about a "choking" episode actually describe what our medical team would consider to be *true* choking. Let's look at an example:

> My baby is 6 months old and showing all the signs of readiness for solids. We gave her a piece of avocado last night and she choked. She was coughing so hard, turning red, and retching so much she threw up and the piece came out and it was huge. We're only giving her purees now, so she won't choke again.
>
> **—Jessica**

While this experience was definitely scary for Jessica, this sounds very much like a baby who was figuring out how to move a piece of avocado around in the mouth and ended up gagging, albeit very hard. But gagging is a normal protective response, as we'll explain in more detail in a moment. And throwing up, though not ideal, isn't unsafe and tells us the food was most likely not in the airway. We'll circle back to this example later, but it's important to first point out that choking is not gagging.

Choking Versus Gagging

Many parents mistakenly think that when a baby gags—which is a common and natural response when learning to eat solid food—that baby is choking. Let's clear up the confusion. Gagging is a natural protective reflex that results in the contraction of the back of the throat, a mechanism that actually protects us from choking.[20] Just like the reflexive kick that occurs when the doctor taps your knee in just the right spot, the gag happens automatically, initiating a rhythmic bottom-up contraction of your pharynx and esophagus (the tube that leads to your stomach) to assist in bringing food up, closing the airway, and stopping the swallowing reflex from making our bodies try to swallow. Gagging is not choking, and gagging does not lead to choking.

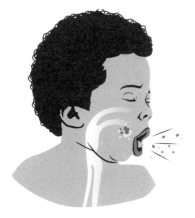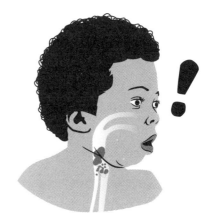

A baby who is gagging (left) *opens the mouth, cups the tongue, and may cough or wretch. A baby who is choking* (right) *typically has open eyes with a look of panic, there is tugging in the neck, and is making high-pitch sounds or no sound.*

When baby gags, you will most likely notice them opening their mouth and making a retching motion, as though they are about to vomit. Baby may lift the sides of their tongue into a cupped or trough shape and stick out their tongue, drool, make a retching noise, cough, cry, or not make much noise at all. Baby will hold their breath each time they gag, but if you listen closely, even a quiet baby will take a breath in after each gag. Baby may look frightened or upset, though many babies are not particularly bothered by gagging.

Gagging is expected as baby learns to chew and eat. However, if you notice that baby is gagging at most meals after a few months of practice, if baby becomes very upset after gagging and it's hard to continue a meal, or if baby is frequently vomiting when eating, we recommend you speak with your child's healthcare provider regarding a referral to an infant feeding and swallowing specialist.

In contrast, choking is generally silent, indicating that no air is flowing into or out of the airway, or baby may make high-pitched noises indicating that they are having trouble breathing. If baby is crying or coughing, this is a good sign that air is flowing in and out of their airway and they are able to breathe. In true choking incidents, baby will appear panicked or terrified and they may look to you for help. If baby has lighter-colored skin, the skin around their mouth and nose may appear purple or blue, though if baby's skin is a darker color, you might not notice a color change. Baby may go limp or unresponsive, which is a clear indication that they are choking, and immediate intervention is needed.

What Exactly Is Choking?

The body has two tubes in the throat: a food tube (esophagus) and an air tube (trachea). These two tubes run right next to each other and as food or liquid passes from the back of the throat to the food tube, it passes the opening of the air tube. If an object or piece of food accidentally enters the wrong pipe and gets stuck in the air tube (or forms a plug over the opening), choking can occur. Choking, by definition, is the full or partial blockage of the airway. Choking typically requires outside intervention such as abdominal thrusts or back slaps to force air out to clear the obstruction. If that all sounds alarming, know these three physiological facts:

1 The body is designed to protect itself from choking.

2 The body has mechanisms to push food into the esophagus, thereby keeping it out of the airway.

3 If an object or food does get near or into the airway, the body is quite effective at getting it out well before it enters or can get stuck in the airway.

How the Body Protects Itself

When baby first starts learning to chew, their body protects itself from choking in the simplest way: by keeping food forward in the

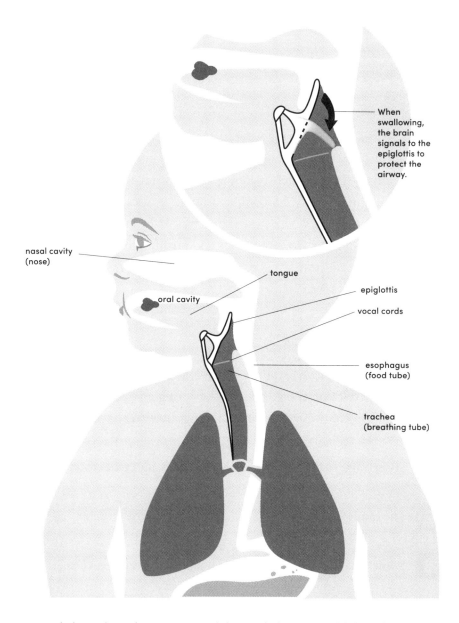

When swallowing, the brain signals to the epiglottis to protect the airway.

nasal cavity (nose)

tongue

oral cavity

epiglottis

vocal cords

esophagus (food tube)

trachea (breathing tube)

Our bodies are designed to protect against choking. As food moves toward the back of the throat, the brain signals to the epiglottis, which folds over the airway to protect it as food moves down the esophagus and into the belly.

mouth, well away from the throat and airway. The body does this with oral motor reflexes and anatomy that make movement of an object toward the back of the mouth and throat particularly challenging. If the food does manage to move too far backward toward the throat, the gag reflex kicks in to close the airway and push the food back out as a second line of defense. If the food does not come to the front of the mouth or out of the mouth at that point, baby's body will prioritize swallowing the food—even if it's unchewed—again closing off the airway and swiftly sending the food down toward the stomach. Should swallowing fail (meaning the coordinated movements don't happen in a timely fashion), and liquid or food gets into the back of the throat anywhere near the airway, baby tends to cough, forcefully expelling air from the lungs and pushing the item up and out. But, despite all these layers of defense, choking occasionally still does happen at all ages.[21]

So How Does Choking Occur, Then?

True choking happens when there is a miscoordination of swallowing and the food (or object) goes down the wrong pipe and gets stuck. For true choking to occur, a number of things have to go wrong:

1 Something makes it past baby's gag and cough reflexes.

2 The brain fails to close off the airway during the swallow.

3 Something lodges in the airway, unable to be coughed out.

Our body's defenses against choking are incredibly powerful, but they are not perfect. Remember, the breathing tube and the food tube are close to one another, and when we swallow, food and liquids must pass the entrance to the breathing tube on the way to the stomach. While the breathing tube is supposed to close on multiple levels (the breathing tube has several doors that close and more than one way to keep itself clear) as the food or liquid moves past it, occasionally there is a disruption and one or more of the anatomical doors fail to fully close at the right time, resulting in choking or aspiration.

Choking is deeply linked to our need to breathe. Breathing is essential and it needs to happen often, and our brain and body prioritize breathing above nearly all other functions. In order to breathe, our airway must be open. Yet every time we swallow, we need to momentarily pause our breathing and close the door to the airway to prevent any food or liquid from going in. Occasionally, our body makes mistakes, and we try to breathe at the same time our body should be closing the breathing tube, which can allow the item to get near the entrance to the airway or even pull food or liquid inside. We cough, usually intensely in response, and typically this is enough to clear whatever is there. But if an item gets lodged in the breathing tube such that our cough reflex is not sufficient to push it out, that item gets stuck and choking occurs. This miscoordination of the swallowing mechanism is surprisingly rare with solids in healthy individuals.

Disruptions to normal swallowing typically occur when the coordination between breathing and swallowing is impacted by moving around, laughing, crying, gasping, or yelling while food or an item is in the mouth. These disruptions will lead to momentary gagging, coughing, and struggle but typically resolve without any extra support from someone else. If a person has something just the right size and shape in the mouth and the need or desire to take a breath (especially a forceful one) happens at the same time they attempt to swallow, the item may get pulled into the breathing tube and get stuck, requiring emergency assistance from someone else.

Now that you have a better understanding of swallowing, gagging, and choking, let's look back at Jessica's email:

> She was coughing so hard, turning red, and retching so much she threw up and a huge piece came out.

Immediately, we are reassured because baby was coughing. Coughing means air is flowing through the airway—baby can't cough if something is stuck in their airway. Retching occurs in tandem with gagging, so it's likely that baby was gagging and coughing very hard, causing the body to throw up. Distressing, yes. Dangerous, no. When a person throws up, the airway naturally closes to keep the acidic contents of the stomach out of the lungs. This allows stomach content to move back up through the food tube into the mouth. If the piece of avocado was thrown up, this alone tells us that it was not inside the airway but instead in the food tube, in the back of the throat, or inside the mouth before it came out.

Now let's dive into a couple more examples:

Hi there. My baby is 8 months and we've been giving solid food since she turned 6 months. Tonight, she had a soft-cooked sweet potato wedge, and I watched her get a piece off, go to swallow and she went into a full choke for the first time since starting solids. Panicked look and she went silent. Thankfully when I pulled her out of her high chair and leaned her forward it came out of her mouth. It has left me very shaken and I'm honestly dreading feeding her. I'm just not sure how to move forward safely. I'm tempted to move to purees and mashes for a while. HELP!

—Shayna

My 16mo was eating a thin triangle piece of watermelon at a birthday party. I looked over at his face and I could tell immediately he was choking. I grabbed him from the high chair and he made a really awful sound and his mouth was wide open and then he went silent. I flipped him over and started back thrusts. I turned him face up and his lips were blue/purple. I slid my finger in from his cheek to see if I could scoop anything out, but his mouth was empty, and he was still silent/ mouth wide open, so I flipped him back over and did back thrusts again. After the second round I flipped him back over and saw the piece of watermelon fall out of the side of his mouth and he finally cried. It all happened fast and was incredibly scary. I'm so grateful to you and your work that I knew what to do and could save him.

—Holly

Both of these parents were terrified. Yet only Holly's story reflects a true choking event. Thankfully, in Holly's instance, the parent was trained in first aid and able to respond appropriately and swiftly.

Let's take a closer look. In Shayna's email, she writes,

> Thankfully when I pulled her out of her high chair and leaned her forward it came out of her mouth.

In this example, the food fell out of her mouth simply by positioning baby to lean forward. In other words, the food was likely never stuck in baby's airway. If it was, it would not have been able to fall from the mouth with a position change. Was the baby struggling with the food? Most likely. Did the food get near her airway briefly, possibly causing it to close just in case as protection? Maybe! But based on the mechanism of clearance, this was not choking.

Holly's story is different:

> My 16mo . . . made a really awful sound and his mouth was wide open and then he went silent . . . his lips were blue/purple. I slid my finger in from his cheek to see if I could scoop anything out but his mouth was empty, and he was still silent/mouth wide open so I flipped him back over and did back thrusts again. After the second round I flipped him back over and saw the piece of watermelon fall out of the side of his mouth and he finally cried.

This toddler was demonstrating classic signs of choking: this "awful sound"—potentially wheezing—is a sign of air trying to get around an obstruction. Lips turning blue, a sign of a lack of oxygen. Mouth check, no food in the mouth. Child silent. The child required back blows to dislodge the obstruction. This toddler was truly choking. Thankfully, their parent knew exactly what to do. While scary to imagine or even to read, remember this: the child was okay. High-quality choking rescue is very effective.

The goal is to monitor baby while they eat and to prepare food appropriately in order to prevent choking from occurring in the first place, as well as to make sure caregivers are trained in choking first aid. Awareness and preparation count here, because in the instance of choking, swift, high-quality rescue maneuvers matter.

What Is Aspiration?

You may have heard the term "aspiration" and have maybe even seen it used interchangeably with "choking." Aspiration and choking are not the same thing. Aspiration occurs when anything (most typically a liquid) slips past the breathing tube's lines of defense and makes its way into the breathing tube itself or the lungs. For choking to occur, something makes its way into the airway and then gets stuck or cannot be coughed out. We all aspirate sometimes (think of when you've taken a drink too quickly, feel it "go the wrong way," and end up coughing for some time after). Our bodies try to clear the airway, but with liquids, a small amount can still make its way into the lungs. When aspiration occurs on an ongoing basis or in a person with a weakened immune system, serious lung infections can develop.

Preventing Choking

Here are the five most important things a parent or caregiver can do to reduce the risk of choking and choking-related injury:

1. Know when and how to administer choking first aid and CPR.

2. Be sure baby is showing all the readiness signs for solids before starting.

3. Create a safe and calm eating environment.[22]

4. Prepare foods appropriately for age and ability.

5. Build chewing skills early on.[23]

1. Learn to Administer Choking First Aid and CPR

While choking is uncommon, it is serious, and if it occurs, you need to act fast. Choking is very responsive to appropriate intervention, and you will very likely save your child's life if you know what to do. Obstruction of the airway can lead to permanent brain damage or death, so it is extremely important that choking first aid is administered quickly and effectively. If you believe a baby or child is choking (not gagging, coughing, retching, or simply frustrated), it's important to jump into action.

Make sure that you and all caregivers know how to perform infant rescue. While there are lots of videos online on how to perform these maneuvers, make sure you also take an in-person class so that you can practice with supervision and receive feedback from the instructor.

In the back of the book are organizations that offer first aid resources. Consider printing them out and posting them on your wall for a visual reference, but remember that this material is not a substitute for certified training. Get trained in choking first aid and infant and child CPR.

Do You Need a Choking Device?

The LifeVac and the Dechoker are two examples of commercial manual suction devices that aim to relieve airway obstruction. If you purchase one of these devices, be sure to still learn infant choking rescue (back blows, chest thrusts, and abdominal thrusts) and infant CPR. These rescue procedures are your first line of defense in the rare event that a child chokes on food or another object. Even if you own and use an airway clearance device, it is crucial to complete pediatric first aid training. These devices are not meant to replace choking first aid but rather act as an intervention when traditional choking first aid measures have failed. As the research is still evolving, there is no right or wrong answer to the question of whether the average family should have one of these devices. Do what works best for you and your family, and make sure the device is the right size/weight for your baby or child.

2. Wait for Readiness Signs

Simply waiting for baby to show the readiness signs we describe in Chapter 7 is the first step in reducing choking risk. If baby does not have these developmental skills, they will have a more challenging time protecting their airway while exploring food. None of the next steps will be as effective if baby does not have developmental readiness for starting solids.

3. Create a Safe Environment

Setting up a safe eating environment is one of the most important things you can do to decrease choking risk. Consider the following:

Before the Meal

- Properly position baby in a completely upright high chair or another appropriate alternative, like sitting securely on your lap. Don't let baby move around while eating. For more on high chairs and other seating, see Chapter 8.
- When we say upright, we mean it. Slouching, slumping, or leaning over can make it more difficult for baby to breathe comfortably, which can increase the likelihood of an uncoordinated swallow. Do not recline baby. Reclining sets

gravity against baby's ability to keep the food at the front of the mouth, where it belongs for learning to chew.[24]

- Remove stray items from the table before mealtime, including wrappers, bottle caps, and so on.
- Practice opening and closing the straps on baby's high chair so you are familiar with them and can quickly remove them if needed.

During the Meal

- Stay within an arm's reach of baby during all meals and snacks.
- Always use high chair straps to keep baby securely in their seat. Falls from the high chair can cause injury, and falling or attempting to climb out of the seat with food in the mouth can cause choking.
- Let baby feed themself. Self-feeding decreases choking risk. Putting food in baby's mouth has been such a large part of infant feeding for so long, it's often assumed to be safe, but this couldn't be further from the truth. Remember, when the body sees food, smells food, touches food, and consciously moves food toward the mouth, the brain begins to prepare the body to swallow.
- Minimize distractions as best you can while baby eats solid food, and maintain a calm environment. We want baby to focus on the food and gather as much information about it as possible before it goes in the mouth, which prepares their brain to manage that food and is the first step in safely swallowing. Distractions can also cause baby to lean over or twist or try to stand in their chair, or lead to gasping, laughing, or crying while eating.
- If baby begins laughing, crying, or throwing their head back, offer a soothing word or tap the tray to bring baby's

attention back to the food. If needed, remove any food on their tray until they are calm.

- If they are crying with food in their mouth, use a soothing voice and a gentle but confident touch to reassure the baby and help them calm down so they can continue to chew or spit out the food. If needed, carefully pick them up to help calm them down.

- Never put your fingers in baby's mouth. While it can be tempting to try to pull a piece of food out of baby's mouth if you see that baby is struggling, putting your fingers in baby's mouth can have the unintended consequence of pushing the item farther back, past baby's natural protective mechanisms, and can lead to choking. Keep in mind, you cannot pull food out of baby's airway if they truly are choking. Anatomically our fingers can't do this. Only choking-rescue procedures can.

- Avoid challenging-to-chew foods when baby is sick, congested, or coughing. Soft, easily mashed foods or purees are a great option when baby is sick.

- Avoid tickling baby while the child is eating or purposefully trying to make them laugh.

While On the Go

- Avoid giving baby chewable foods when you are driving.
- Do not offer food to baby in a moving stroller. The motion increases risk, and most strollers are not positioned upright enough to be safe for eating.
- Teach baby that they must sit down while eating. Even if they are not in a high chair, we want them to learn early that they must always be seated when food is in their mouth. You can remove the food from baby's hands if needed and help get their body into a seated position in a chair, on your

lap, or on the floor if their high chair is unavailable. Infants who learn this rule from the start grow into toddlers who automatically sit down whenever they are offered food at a party or at school.

Now, is it possible to always be sitting in a supportive chair, in a calm quiet environment, without the sniffles, and never making any noise, crying, or laughing? Absolutely not. But we can use this information wisely when selecting what we serve, when, and how. Instead of avoiding certain foods, turn your attention to the environment in which food is consumed.

Lastly, remember that, during infancy, fatal choking incidents are more likely to occur from nonfood objects, not food. Regularly get down on the floor to view your home from baby's eye level and pick up objects (or fallen pieces of food) that pose a risk, so they are out of sight and out of reach.

Nonfood Objects and Choking

While it is rare for an infant to die by choking, the data shows that choking deaths due to nonfood objects are more prevalent than those from food. And the data also suggests that this risk from nonfood objects doesn't go away after baby becomes a toddler. While a toddler who has learned to chew through early practice will likely be safer at the table, they are now mobile and are constantly encountering new and interesting objects, not all of them safe. They walk, they run, they pick up objects, they put objects in their mouth, and they keep moving. Recent data also shows that around 50 percent of choking-related deaths in young children on average do not involve food but objects that may include everyday household items such as stickers, marbles, balloons, coins, and small toys.[25,26] That is why it is important to regularly get down on the floor to view your home from baby's eye level and put away any food and objects that pose a risk, so they are out of sight and out of reach.

4. Prepare Foods Appropriately

Parents and medical professionals alike tend to worry most about the food: What foods should we avoid? What textures are safest? Is the food a choking hazard? Based on the data, common choking hazards tend to have the following characteristics:

- **x** Small
- **x** Firm or springy
- **x** Slippery
- **x** Round or tapered

You can share almost any food that you eat with baby as long as it is modified to meet baby's age and developmental ability, so baby can easily and effectively pick the food up and get it to their mouth. This is done by reducing the factors just listed that make a food more likely to get stuck in the airway: size, shape, consistency, and so on. In Part 3, we'll talk about specific sizes and shapes for the different developmental stages of baby's solid food journey, but in general, it makes sense to avoid giving infants foods like candy (aka high-choking-risk foods with minimal nutritional value). When it comes to the many nutritious foods that naturally have characteristics that increase choking risk, we don't want you to avoid these, but they do require some modification to be safer. As you introduce solid food, download the Solid Starts App to look up suggestions on how to cut and safely prepare any food for a child's age and developmental ability.

Choking Risk Versus Choking Hazards

While we know that there are characteristics of food that increase choking risk, looking only at the specific texture of a food does not give us the whole picture. Certain foods come up again and again in the published literature as common causes of choking, and these foods often share some or all of the characteristics that heighten choking risk. But not all food-related cases of choking involve these common choking hazards. This makes it clear that, although rare, an individual hypothetically can choke on any food at any time in their life. And it suggests that something else is going on that also contributes to choking risk. This other, often overlooked "something else" is the feeding environment and circumstances we just discussed. And it turns out that the environment and circumstances are the most important contributing factors for choking risk and the most easily addressed.[27,28] This means that a child sitting at a table eating a whole grape while supervised by a caregiver is generally safer than a child who is running around with minimal supervision while eating a food that we would all consider "safe."

In our clinical work, we have cared for a few children who survived a choking incident, and while some might look at these anecdotes and focus on the specific foods consumed, we also see the environment and the role it played in these tragic moments. One child was riding his bicycle in his house while eating whole grapes. Another child threw a grape in the air and tried to catch it with his mouth. We have also cared for a child who choked on mini marshmallows after opening a bag while at the supermarket, stuffed too many in their mouth, and accidentally inhaled one. Tragedies like these are uncommon, but when they happen, they have devastating results for children and families.

While one approach is to warn all parents to avoid grapes and mini marshmallows, the reality is most toddlers and young children will be exposed to a high-risk food or a high-risk environment as they grow and eat more meals outside the home. Choking risk is a constant throughout our lives. We believe that focusing on the environment and what we *can* control will make a difference.

5. Build Skills for Safer Eating

You know by now that building the skills to safely eat real food takes time and lots of practice. But this period of baby's life is the ideal time for them to instinctively fumble through learning these skills because of strong protective mechanisms and an intense drive to bring things to their own mouth and explore. And as the data shows, death by choking is an incredibly rare occurrence in infancy and toddlerhood, and the risk is low when you make the environment safe and prepare foods to match baby's development. As you and baby do this work, try to keep this knowledge at the front of your mind.

Every opportunity to explore food at the table helps baby build their chewing coordination and their oral sensory awareness, also known as the "mental map" of the inside of their own mouth, or the ability to know where all the parts of the mouth are in relation to each other. As an adult, you know what's going on inside your mouth even though you can't see inside it. You can feel where any food is and know if it's fully chewed or not. You can even tell if there's a tiny eggshell in your scrambled eggs, carefully find that eggshell with your tongue, and politely spit it out without having to spit out the whole bite of food.

That level of sensory awareness takes years to fully develop, and constant touch and pressure exposure when baby is most eager to do so helps lay the foundations. Every time baby explores food in their mouth, their mental map gets filled in a little bit more clearly. As this happens, eating becomes more successful and safer.[29]

Summary

✓ Contrary to popular belief, choking is *not* a common cause of death in babies and children.

✓ Babies don't need teeth to eat real food. They can munch and grind with their gums.

✓ Letting babies feed themselves reduces the risk of choking.

✓ Many parents confuse gagging for choking, so it's important to learn the difference.

✓ Keep choking risk low by creating a calm eating environment and modifying foods as needed.

✓ Take a course that includes choking first aid. Even though the risk is low, response time matters and it is essential for all caregivers to know infant choking rescue.

Part Three

Building Skill

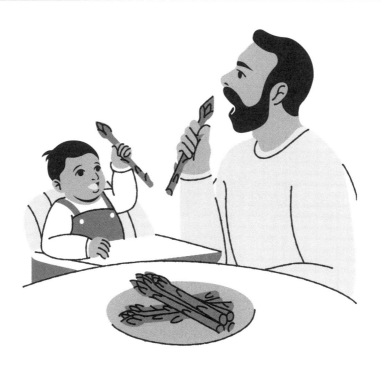

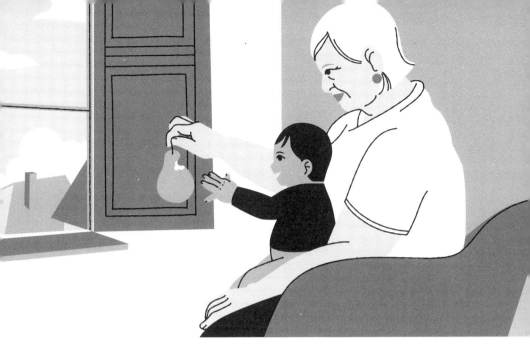

Chapter Seven

Is Baby Ready for Solids?

Our baby Lucy is a happy, healthy baby. At our 4-month appointment, our pediatrician told us she was ready for solid food, so we tried. She couldn't sit up well so we reclined her chair so she could keep her head and neck straight. But she had no interest in eating and just kept trying to turn away from us. What are we doing wrong?

—Solomon

We are not surprised that Solomon's baby didn't take to solid food at first. Unable to sit upright or even hold her head steady, she was simply not ready to be starting solid food. So why did her doctor recommend she start?

Over the years, recommendations for when to introduce solid food have changed dramatically, and there hasn't always been alignment in the medical community—until recently. Today, major medical authorities now agree: it's best to wait to introduce solid food until baby shows all of the signs that they are *developmentally* ready.[1,2]

For most full-term babies, this will be around 6 months of age, though some are ready a bit earlier and some a few weeks later.[3] All of these scenarios are normal. Instead of watching the calendar and waiting for baby to turn a certain age, look for these signs of developmental readiness:

1 **Sits with minimal support while holding the head up.** At a minimum, baby should to be able to sit completely upright (such as in a high chair or on your lap) and be able to maintain their head upright. These two things are critical for chewing and swallowing safety. If baby needs to be reclined to be stable, they are not ready.

2 **Brings a hand to mouth while sitting upright.** This movement indicates that baby is strong enough to bring food to their own mouth. This is a critical skill in safe eating, as we discussed in Chapter 6, as self-feeding in and of itself decreases the risk of choking.

3 **Shows interest in food and/or what you are eating.** If baby is not yet interested in what you are eating or lacks interest in food offered to them, meals can become a battle of wills. Baby is ready to explore solid food when you see that they are noticing food that you eat, watching you eat, and expressing interest in your food or utensil.

There is no need to formally assess baby for these signs. All you need to do is keep an eye out as these skills emerge during playtime and while baby is watching you eat your meals. If baby is not showing these signs by 7 months of age, it's a good idea to check in with your doctor or healthcare provider, who may recommend some support from a specialist who can help baby progress.

What Does Sitting with Minimal Support Look Like?

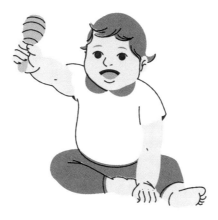

Baby is able to hold their head and neck upright without slouching when seated in a high chair or on an adult's lap, and baby is able to reach for something and bring it to their mouth.

It's okay if baby can't sit by themselves on the floor, and it's okay if baby can't get in and out of the seated position independently. What matters is that baby is strong enough to sit upright with the support of a high chair or on an adult's lap. Watch baby's control of the head and neck. Stability is crucial; as long as baby can keep the head and body upright for several minutes in the high chair or on your lap, they are strong enough to explore solid food. But if baby needs support holding the head upright and steady, consider waiting a week or two and try again.

Readiness and Prematurity

For most healthy preterm babies, we suggest looking for the signs that they are ready to start solids around 6 months *chronological* age, assuming that most (not necessarily all) premature babies are ready sometime between 6 months chronological age and 6 months adjusted (or corrected) age.

For babies born prior to 32 weeks gestation or babies with other co-occurring or underlying medical conditions or developmental differences, we strongly recommend you consult with your medical and therapy teams to better assess when baby is ready and if they would benefit from additional support or modifications. For infants born very premature, such as those born before 30 weeks gestation, there is some research to suggest that solids should not be introduced prior to 3 months adjusted or corrected age, even if baby is at 6+ months chronological age.[4,5] In general, signs of developmental readiness are more important than age, but for some babies with medical needs, adaptations may be necessary to ensure that they are given opportunities to explore food in a safe manner before 12 months of age.

Unwinding the Myths about Starting Solids

You may have heard some of the common myths about starting solids that are still floating around, maybe from your doctor or your family or parenting forums. From inaccurate readiness signs to using solids as a quick fix for a variety of challenges in infancy, many of these myths are passed around so often that they seem true. Unfortunately, starting solids is sometimes offered up as a "Band-Aid" for a variety of difficult situations that come up with young babies, including bottle- and breastfeeding issues, disrupted sleep, and other normal yet tough parts of parenting. To cut through any noise, we're listing some of those myths here. If they sound at all familiar, you'll be reassured to know that they have no basis in science.

Myth

You need to wait for the tongue thrust to go away before you start solids.

Remember those protective mechanisms young babies have? If you've ever seen something touch a young baby's lips or tongue and then seen the tongue dart out in response, you've observed the tongue thrust reflex at work. Historically, some medical professionals have wrongfully assumed that if baby's tongue thrust is still intact, they are not ready to start solids because the tongue will move the food right back out of the mouth. First, there's no research to back this up, or to show that the tongue thrust reflex is somehow dangerous if present when starting solids, or that a baby will be more prepared to learn to eat solids if this reflex has disappeared. If you are spoon-feeding purees, the tongue thrust will likely make things a bit more messy as the food gets pushed out, but if you introduce a baby to finger foods while this reflex is intact, the tongue movement helps babies naturally learn how to spit food out. What's more, the tongue thrust also helps them lick, taste, and explore foods that they bring to their lips. Even after the reflex goes away, it's still a very well-practiced motion that babies will do anyway, so it would be nearly impossible to avoid.

Myth

Baby needs teeth before they can be offered chewable food.

As we've discussed, it is a misconception that babies need teeth to eat. In fact, the teeth humans use to chew (our molars) don't come in until after baby's first birthday. Babies can munch and break down food quite successfully with their gums, tongue, and palate, and there is a lack of research to suggest that babies are less capable managing solid foods without teeth.

Myth

Breast milk and formula aren't enough.

Breast milk and formula provide all of baby's nutrition in the first 6 months of life and continue to be the main source of nutrition until baby has the skills to chew and swallow enough solid food—a skill that can take months to hone. Introducing solids in a low-pressure way that does not emphasize volume allows baby to practice the skills of eating without displacing breast milk or formula. In later infancy, usually around 9+ months and up, many babies start to consume more significant amounts of solids, which help meet the older infant's shifting nutritional needs, such as their need for iron. By 12 to 15 months, when most of their nutrition will come from solid foods, they'll be ready, willing, and happy to eat to their belly's content.

Myth

If baby needs to gain weight, you should start solids early.

Some medical professionals continue to recommend that if a baby is not gaining weight properly from breast milk or formula alone, they should start solid food, even if baby is not developmentally ready for solids. We also hear of medical providers encouraging families of babies who are developmentally ready to start finger foods but who are not gaining weight well on breast milk or infant formula to start pureed foods to help baby gain weight. The problem with this is that it doesn't address the root cause of the issue—breast- or bottle-feeding challenges or underlying medical conditions. Most young babies do not have the skills to get a wide variety of solid food in the belly right away to make up for their challenges with breast- or bottle-feeding.

And for those who do get a good amount of purees swallowed, it can further displace breast milk or formula, whose nutritional diversity and caloric density is often more optimal than purees, and it further delays baby's exposure to finger foods.

If baby is struggling with weight gain before the introduction of solids, it's highly possible that there is a solvable medical reason, such as oral motor challenges, frequency of feeds, or digestive discomfort. Rather than jumping to try to fix the issue by serving purees and starting solids early, it's best to work with a medical professional to determine if referrals to specialists (such as a lactation consultant, pediatric occupational therapist or speech-language pathologist, pediatric dietitian, or pediatric gastroenterologist) are needed to help identify and address the underlying reason for poor weight gain.

Myth

Starting solids will help baby sleep through the night.

While it may seem logical that if a baby's belly is fuller with solid food they will sleep better, the research does not show that solid food measurably improves infant sleep.[6] A baby who consumes more during the day (solids and/or breast milk or formula) may be less likely to feed during the night, but night waking does not tend to decrease with solid food intake. In fact, starting solids may disrupt sleep as baby's gut gets used to it all, especially if they are encouraged to eat large enough amounts to prevent hunger at night. Gas and changes in the consistency and frequency of bowel movements are all commonly associated with starting solids and can also disrupt sleep.

Myth

Starting solids early helps babies with reflux.

Certain pediatric healthcare providers may suggest starting solids early around 4 months of age to help with infant reflux; however, the research does not support this. About half of infants have reflux, and most babies tend to be "happy spitters," where no intervention is needed. Reflux tends to peak around 4 months of age and resolve on its own around 12 months of age as baby's digestive anatomy becomes more mature.[7,8,9] Starting solids early does not appear to improve reflux or make it resolve sooner. If baby's reflux symptoms are causing discomfort, treatments like changes in infant formula, removing milk from mom's diet, and certain acid-reducing medications may be recommended by a doctor or healthcare provider. Other interventions such as addressing constipation, avoiding overfeeding, holding baby upright after feeds, burping frequently, and making sure baby's diaper isn't too tight, can also help relieve some reflux-related discomfort.

Myth
Offering baby a variety of purees early will expand their palate (aka "taste training").

Some say that you can train baby's taste buds through early exposure. While variety and repeated exposure to different flavors is an important way to expand baby's palate once they are ready for solids, "taste training" before baby is developmentally ready for solids does not appear to have extra benefits and is likely to backfire. Acceptance of foods is about much more than just flavor. Chewing practice, the feeling of being in control of eating, and the ability to easily push food back out of the mouth when needed are what help babies and toddlers accept a variety of foods. The research has found that it is variety and repeated exposure to foods over time that builds tolerance and acceptance.[10]

Starting Solids Before Baby Is Ready

There is no need to begin solids before baby is ready unless baby is at high risk of food allergies, in which case your doctor or healthcare provider may recommend introducing certain food allergens (particularly peanut and/or egg) at 4 months of age in a puree, powder, or liquid form. Research and recommendations on food allergy introduction are rapidly evolving, and in Chapter 14 we discuss the importance of early and sustained food allergen exposure.

If you need to start solids before developmental readiness, it is safest to offer very small amounts of purees. Offering chewable foods before baby can stay upright and self-feed is not recommended, as placing food in baby's mouth has been shown to increase the risk of choking,[11,12] and baby needs head and neck control, along with the ability to sit with minimal support, to safely swallow and coordinate the use of the muscles in the tongue and mouth.[13,14]

Keep in mind, feeding baby larger volumes of solid food before they are ready can lead to negative outcomes:

Starting solids too early can strain baby's relationship with food and their caregivers.

A concern with introducing solids before baby is ready is that the child's interest in eating may not be there just yet. In this scenario, pushing baby to taste food they have no interest in can stress a child's relationship with their caregivers and create a negative association with food, their high chair, and mealtime. As we discussed in Parts 1 and 2 of the book, listening to baby's body language and communication is critical, so showing interest in food and mealtimes truly matters. When babies are started on solids too early and pressured to taste foods (whether purees or chewable food), it can result in feeding challenges and food refusal for months and even years to come.

Introducing food before baby can sit up and self-feed increases choking risk and can cause food-refusal behavior.

When you start solids before baby is able to sit upright or self-feed, they will not have the stability in their core muscles necessary to support the important fine motor movements in their mouth and throat needed to easily move food (even if it's purees) back toward the throat to safely swallow. Babies who are not ready to handle solids often shut down and refuse to participate if offered more than small tastes. If pushed and pressured, most babies will eventually get upset and cry at mealtimes. Not only can this quickly spiral into more persistent refusal, but crying with food in the mouth can be dangerous—increasing the risk of aspiration (food entering the airway) or choking. The brain can more easily trip up the wires when baby is frustrated, upset, and not in control of their body or the food.

In some cultures, babies are offered tastes of food enjoyed by the rest of the family as early as 1 month of age. While an occasional lick or small taste for fun and tradition is generally okay as long as baby is a willing participant, we encourage you to review Chapter 9 to learn which foods are safe for infants and which you should avoid.

Following Doctor's Orders

A doctor may advise introducing purees around 4 months of age for various reasons, including food allergy prevention, which we discuss in detail in Chapter 14. If you decide to start solids before baby is showing the signs of readiness, follow these tips:

- Offer just small tastes (a dab on the tip of your finger or a small spoonful) to avoid overwhelming baby or displacing breast milk or formula intake.

- Feed responsively: hold the spoon (or your finger with food on it) within reach of baby, then let them open their mouth, lean in, and accept it. If baby can reach out and grab the utensil or finger, even better.
- Stop offering solid food if baby loses interest (pulling or turning head away, crying, arching back, etc.).
- Consider positioning baby sitting on your lap with your body fully supporting them. Do not recline a baby when they eat.

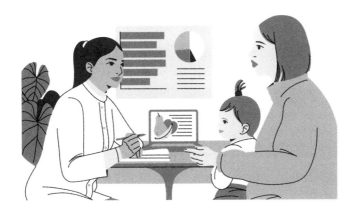

When the Doctor Says to Start Solids Early

Just as it was confusing for baby Lucy's dad, Solomon, it can be confusing when your doctor says to start solids before baby is ready. The topic often comes up at a baby's 4-month well-child visit to the doctor, and unfortunately, many healthcare providers still suggest the outdated practice of starting solids at that time, without considering developmental skills.

If you find yourself in this scenario, consider asking your doctor the following questions:

 What is my baby doing developmentally that makes you feel they are ready?

2 What is the benefit of my baby starting solids at this age?

3 Are you recommending solid food for my baby for a specific reason, or is this a recommendation you make to most of your patients?

While it can be uncomfortable to ask additional questions of baby's medical provider, most want to be sure their patients understand their recommendations and expect questions, and the answers are important to help you make an informed decision about how to proceed. If their answers do not seem in line with what you have learned and you feel up to it, you can also ask if you can review the World Health Organization, American Academy of Family Physicians, and/or American Academy of Pediatrics recommendations with your physician.[15,16] Keep in mind that your medical practitioner is constantly learning, and this could be an excellent time to discuss what your plans are for baby and open up a dialogue. That being said, you can also simply collect their additional thoughts on the three preceding questions and thank them, then use your own judgment to make the decision that feels right for you.

The Magic of 6 to 8 Months

If you've been reading this book from page 1, you've already gotten a deep primer on all the ways that starting solids at 6 months supports baby and fits right into their natural development stage. If you've flipped to this section to get right to the nitty-gritty, we encourage you to read Chapter 3, which underlines the reasons why we believe so strongly in the benefits of starting solids during the magic window and all of the reasons this approach can help baby learn to chew, build a joyous relationship with food, develop confidence and trust, and join you at meals as an active participant.

Summary

✓ Start looking for signs that baby is ready to start solids around 6 months of age.

✓ Signs of readiness include (1) sitting with minimal support while holding the head and neck with stability; (2) ability to bring at least one hand to the mouth; and (3) interest in food.

✓ Starting solids too soon can be unsafe and compromise baby's relationship with food and you.

✓ Review the evidence and unwind the myths before you make your choices. There is a lot of misinformation floating around, and understanding the landscape will help you ask questions.

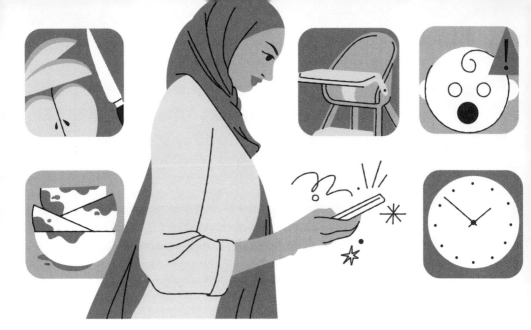

Chapter Eight

Practical Preparation for Getting Started

I am pregnant and my sister, who is a nurse, suggested I take a CPR class before starting solids. And one of my friends told me I need a baby food blender and a certain type of high chair so baby doesn't choke. I am now feeling really overwhelmed. What are all the things I need to do and get before giving my baby solid food?

—Val, mom-to-be

This chapter is your guide to preparing so that when baby is ready to start solids, you are, too. Our first piece of advice: don't worry too much about gear. Much, if not most of it, is unnecessary. Food can be prepared with the basic cooking equipment you already own—you do not need special baby food steamers, blenders, or mesh feeders. And when it comes to mealtime, food can go directly on the high chair tray or table (plates and bowls will be tipped over anyway) and baby can eat directly with their hands (and we recommend you let them do so). The only things you really need for those first meals are a firm understanding of infant safety, a safe seating arrangement, and realistic expectations.

Safety Education

While choking is uncommon, educating yourself and any other adults who will be taking care of baby is a must. All caretakers need to know:

1 How to spot the difference between gagging and choking.

2 How to perform infant rescue in case of an emergency.

If you have not already, read Chapter 6 before starting solids so you have a firm understanding of gagging and choking and learn how to perform infant rescue. While we recommend you sign up for an in-person class on infant rescue, you can also visit SolidStarts.com to download our free rescue guides, which walk you through the motions in detail.

Safe Seating

The safest place for baby to eat is in an upright, supportive position. While that can be from your lap or in certain positions on the floor if needed, a high chair is the most practical way to safely position baby for meals.

Choosing a High Chair

When you are choosing a high chair, we suggest getting a chair with three key components:

1 **Upright seat.** Look for high chairs that have a totally upright seat. If they have reclining features, don't use them when feeding.

2 **Adjustable foot plate.** Look for a chair that enables baby's feet to be firmly planted on a foot plate with the knees bent at a 90-degree angle. This position puts baby's trunk, pelvis, and lower body in the most optimal position for eating.[1]

3 **Removable tray.** If you have a dining table, it's great to be able to bring baby's chair right up to the table with you from the beginning so they can watch you eat and be part of mealtime. Babies learn best by watching you and feeling engaged with a trusted caregiver.[2,3] When baby watches a trusted caregiver, the mirror neurons in their brain fire, encouraging babies to copy our movements. Watching you eat will be key to learning.

Do High Chairs Need a Footrest?

A footrest that baby can bear weight on or push their feet into helps baby get into an optimal position for chewing and swallowing.[4,5] Here's why: the muscles in our mouth are really small and do very specialized, careful work. To help them do these super specialized movements, we need to give them a strong, stable base. Think of the last meal you had on a barstool with nowhere to put your feet—not only can it be uncomfortable, it makes it harder for you to remain stable while moving your arms and other small muscles. Some babies eat fine without a supportive footrest, but for others, the additional effort of using more tummy and back muscles makes eating a bit too challenging to enjoy.

For a review of current high chairs, see our website at SolidStarts.com.

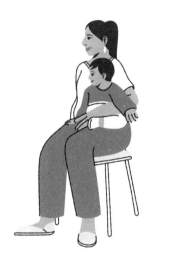 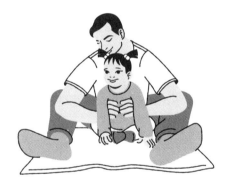

High Chair Alternatives

If a high chair is not in your budget or if you prefer to not use one, here are two options for positioning baby safely for eating:

1 **Seated on your lap.** Position baby's back against your body, keeping one arm wrapped around their waist. Scoot your chair as close to the table as possible with baby facing the

table. If the table is too high for baby in this position, try placing a thick book or pillow underneath your own bottom to raise you and baby a bit higher.

2 **Seated on the floor with you for support.** Sit on the floor and put baby between your legs, letting baby's legs form a "ring" with the bottoms of their feet facing each other. Position baby's back against your body. Support baby's hips with both hands or wrap your arm around their midsection to stabilize them. Use a coffee table, shoebox, or step stool to elevate the food to baby's belly level if you'd like.

How to Position Baby in the High Chair

Proper positioning at mealtime is important for swallowing safety, oral motor movements, and the ability for baby to use their arms and hands.[6] Proper positioning includes the following:

→ Back should be completely upright and straight, shoulders in line with hips.
→ Bent knees with feet planted on a footrest, bench, or other surface for support. You may need to slide baby's bottom slightly forward in the seat to allow them to reach the footrest.
→ Baby's arms should be free, and the table or tray should be below baby's chest level so baby can easily reach forward or even slightly down to pick up food on the tray or table (they should not have to reach up or hunch their shoulders to grab food).

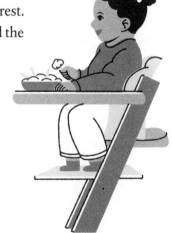

Baby's Back

When baby is strapped into the high chair, look at them from the side. Is their back completely upright? You want to see their shoulders in line with or in front of their hips. If baby is leaning backward, place a rolled towel or small blanket behind their back (from their pelvis to their shoulder blades) to help them sit more upright.

Baby's Feet and Legs

If your high chair has an adjustable footrest, adjust its height and position so baby's feet can touch the footrest, ideally with the ability to bear weight forward into the feet. Take off socks and footie pajamas without grip so baby's feet don't slide on the footrest.

If baby's feet do not reach the footrest, try adding a towel or blanket roll behind their back to help position baby's bottom closer to the front of the seat. Err on the side of having the footrest adjusted too high as opposed to too low.

If you cannot position the footrest to touch baby's feet, use sturdy tape to attach a box, yoga block, or thick book to the footrest. Make sure it is secured so it doesn't slip when baby bears weight into it.

If your chair doesn't have a footrest, you can try to pull a bench, stool, or large packing box up under the high chair. There are products on the market you can purchase to add a footrest to a high chair as well; just search "footrest for high chair" online.

Baby's Arms

Now, look at baby from the front. Can baby's arms easily reach objects on the tray? Some babies may need a little boost under their bottom to be able to functionally use their arms while in the high chair. The tray should be slightly above their belly button, and they should be able to easily rest their arms and hands on the tray or table in front of them. If baby is too low—you see the tray at their chest level—try putting a thick book or firm folded blanket under their bottom to give them a boost. When doing this, always use the safety harness on the high chair.

Always Use the High Chair Harness and Safety Straps

It is estimated that about five thousand infants are evaluated every year in emergency departments in the United States after falling from a high chair.[7,8] High chair systems with straps or harness systems ensure that a child is safe and secure. Always use high chairs as the manufacturer recommends, including properly securing safety straps or harnesses to keep a child safe and secure in their chair.

What if I want to be able to get baby out fast in the event of an emergency?
Using a car seat was probably confusing at the beginning, too, and so was the stroller. After a million uses, it's second nature. Same here. If you feel nervous about getting baby out quickly, practice unbuckling the harness multiple times before your first mealtime so you feel confident that you can operate it swiftly if you need to.

Other Helpful Products

While we are firm believers that as long as baby is in a safe seating arrangement you don't need to buy any special items to feed baby safely, there are a few items that make mealtimes with baby easier and less messy. Here is a list of items to consider:

→ splat mat or way to protect the floor
→ small open cup
→ straw cup
→ small utensils with short handles
→ unbreakable, shallow bowl
→ unbreakable plate with a rim
→ bib, smock, or dark onesies that don't show stains
→ waterproof placemat or way to protect table, if needed
→ washcloths

There are endless options for each of these products online. Know that no one single product will make or break the feeding experience, and every product on the market has its imperfections. Baby plates and bowls that suction to the table will be pulled off and tipped over, bibs will be tugged at, and placemats will be peeled off and thrown. You may also find that the more products you put in front of baby, the more distracted baby can become. Many parents start out buying all the things only to find a couple of weeks in that they are using very few of them. Or that they use them much later in the solids journey when baby is less likely to pull, tip, tug, and throw. For the first couple of weeks of starting solids all you really need is you, baby, food, and a safe place for baby to sit.

Incorporating Solids into Your Day

Good news: you can decide what time of day to offer solid foods based on a mix of what works best for baby and you. Pick a time of day when baby is generally rested and alert. You want baby to have had a bit of time to digest their breast milk or formula, so they don't throw up if they gag, but not be too hungry as to feel impatient. Remember, babies are not hunger-motivated right at first; they are motivated to explore and learn by putting these new "toys" in their mouths. Hangry babies will quickly grow frustrated with solids, as they do not have the eating skills just yet to meet that hunger need.

For many parents, morning is the time baby is well rested, most alert, and eager to learn. Morning is also a great time of day to introduce new foods because if baby has an allergic reaction, there's ample time in the day to observe baby and handle any hospital or doctor visits without losing too much sleep. That said, baby's mealtimes don't have to be at the same time each day at first. Start with one opportunity to explore solid food a day. You can do breakfast during the week and lunch on the weekends. Or breakfast one day and dinner another. Fold the meals into your life however they fit until you find a rhythm that works for you.

Plan to offer breast milk or formula around 30 minutes prior to coming to the table. Baby will likely want breast milk or formula after their mealtime as well, and this is normal. Many babies won't consume much solid food—if anything—when first starting. Remember that baby's primary source of nutrition is still breast milk or formula and to focus on skills, not consumption.

If baby is very sick or having a tough day, you may consider skipping the solid meals for that day to keep their solids experiences positive. Bad congestion can also increase the risk of choking. In these early months of starting solids, it's completely fine if a day or two goes by without offering solid food because you or baby are having a tough day, or it just doesn't work in the schedule. What's most important is that baby enjoys their time at the table and has the interest and stamina to learn.

On this note, don't expect to change anything with breast or bottle feeds for a while. Solids is about learning, not intake, for the first few months, so there will likely be minimal to no decrease in baby's breast milk or formula intake.

Setting Realistic Expectations

If you've never seen a baby eat, you may not know what this is going to look like. Here are a few things to keep in mind to help prepare you for what's to come:

→ Baby may not consume much (if anything) and may only touch or play with the food. This is normal and does not mean you or baby have failed. As long as you are eating in front of baby to show them how it's done, it's still a successful "meal."

→ This will get messy! And it is going to be messy for quite some time. Many parents prepare for mess by putting splat mats under baby's high chair on the floor (a garbage bag cut open to lie flat or a shower curtain liner will work as well) and covering baby with a bib, a smock, or simply a dark-colored onesie that doesn't show stains. Have a lot of washcloths handy as well!

→ Meals may last only 5 to 10 minutes at first before baby fusses. This is normal. The experience is completely new for baby. Sitting upright is tiring for baby at this age, and learning to eat and chew is hard work!

How you show up at the table matters more than any high chair, bib, or plate that you buy. *The most important gear is your attitude.*

One mistake we see many parents make when starting solids is focusing too much on the gear and not enough on the experience. You could make a beautiful meal and serve it on the most fancy baby plate, in the most expensive high chair, but if baby does not want to be at the table with you, none of this will matter. How you show up at the table matters more than any high chair, bib, or plate that you buy.

Make mealtime a place where baby wants to be. Help baby feel that the table is a wonderful, safe, and fun place. Align mealtime with the deep comfort of connection and love, by smiling at baby as they experience the meal, listening to and acknowledging their efforts and communication. Your positive, calm attention will show baby how much you trust them to explore and how much you enjoy watching them learn. These actions—eating with baby, sharing food, and focusing on cultivating a strong connection at meals—all help lay a strong foundation for baby and are also research-backed strategies that can help prevent mealtime issues down the road.[9]

Summary

✓ You do not need special baby food steamers or blenders. Food can be prepared with the basic cooking equipment you already have.

✓ If you have not already taken an infant rescue class, be sure to do so before starting solids.

✓ If you're buying a high chair, get one with an upright seat, adjustable foot plate, and removable tray.

✓ Pay attention to baby's rhythms and daily schedule. When might be a good time to offer them solids? Choose a time when baby is calm, well rested, and not too hungry.

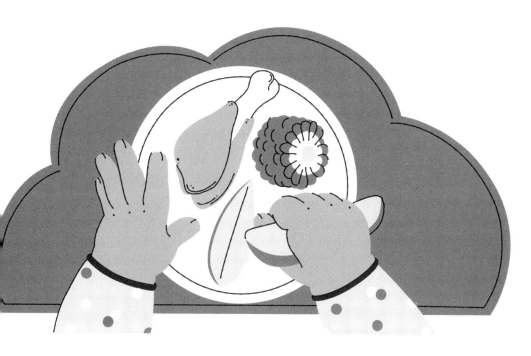

Chapter Nine

First Foods

George's family had a tradition of cooking and eating dinner together on Wednesday nights. They knew this was how they wanted to introduce George to foods at the table for the first time. Once George was ready, they chose a meal of fajitas, which were a family favorite. They prepared the meal, being sure to cut some of the meat and vegetables into thick, long strips that would be easy for George to pick up. For these pieces, they also reduced the seasoning to avoid too much spicy flavor. Carin, his mom, said that sharing this meal with George was something she would never forget.

Almost any food in the world can be served to a baby, and nearly every meal can be baby-friendly as long as you approach each food with an eye to modifying it for baby's development and skill level, so they can pick the food up and eat it themselves. This chapter is all about first foods for baby, and we'll walk you through some great options and how to prepare them in a way that will help baby safely learn to eat.

Small modifications for baby might be needed, and we will explain the basics of how to make sure foods are prepared appropriately for baby's age, but these tweaks will become second nature over time, so unless you are managing allergies, everyone can share and eat the same food—no extra cooking just for baby.

When we do modify food, we are thinking about safety, baby's stage of development, ease of consumption and preparation, and whether the modification supports self-feeding. Not all foods require modification from how you may prepare it for your family, and as you'll learn, the stage of development matters when it comes to preparing food.

Though there can be tremendous pressure from parents, friends, family members, and food companies, you are not obliged in any way to offer baby any particular foods or brands. Let this be an invitation to serve foods that you love and that are accessible to you.

Choose the Foods You Want to Eat

When considering baby's first foods, it can be tempting to focus on "baby food" or on trying to guess what baby will like and successfully eat. Instead, consider flipping this and choose food *you* enjoy, then share a bit of that meal with baby. It is easy to get caught up in baby cookbooks and special meals, but with decades of experience working with families (and raising kids ourselves), what we can say is this: if you want your child to eventually eat what you eat, introduce them to those foods and flavors upfront.

If offering the foods you eat feels too fast or scary for you, pick a food or two that is specifically for baby, then add a bit of it to your own plate too. Many families start with single ingredients, simply prepared for baby, in those first few weeks, then advance to more complex meals with mixed items and a few options later on. This is also fine. Simple foods simply prepared are delicious, too. You can continue to aim for foods you and your family enjoy with the goal of bringing baby into your family's food culture, but it's challenging to model eating a food that you don't enjoy or don't really want to eat.

Foods to Avoid Versus Foods to Modify

Almost any food can be made safe for baby, including some high-risk foods, which is why we devoted an entire chapter to teaching you about age-by-age, developmentally appropriate food preparation. As you'll learn in depth in Chapter 10, you can reduce the risk dramatically by appropriately preparing all foods, including foods that present a high choking risk but are nutritious (like seeds, whole nuts, baby carrots, apples, pomegranate arils, grapes, and more). Despite certain foods' riskier profile, we don't advise fully avoiding them. We recommend modifying them to reduce the choking risk and to allow baby to get familiar with them so they will be more likely to accept them—and eventually learn to eat them in their un-modified form—in toddlerhood.

But even though most foods are safe or can be modified to be safer, some foods should be avoided.

We're starting with this short list to ease your mind, and to show you that, except for these, most foods can be prepared in a way that is safe for baby as soon as they begin solids.

There are two categories of foods to avoid:

- **x** Foods with a high choking risk that cannot be easily modified
- **x** Foods that might make baby sick

Avoid foods that pose a higher risk of choking that cannot be easily modified to reduce risk, such as hard candy, gum, and marshmallows, among many others.

Avoid foods that can make babies sick. Babies do not have fully developed immune systems like adults have and, therefore, are more at risk of developing severe symptoms from foodborne illnesses. Based on U.S. health recommendations, to reduce the likelihood of illness, avoid the following:[1,2,3,4,5,6,7,8]

→ **Honey and honey-based sauces,** because of the increased risk of a rare condition called infant botulism. While this risk primarily impacts the youngest babies, authorities consider honey to be safe after baby's first birthday.

→ **Raw or rare animal proteins,** such as sushi, undercooked seafood, raw or rare meats, and runny eggs. Fully cook all meats, poultry, seafood, and eggs.

→ **Cured and smoked meats and fish,** including deli meats. Many of these pose an increased risk of foodborne illness due to not being fully cooked or due to how they are processed and stored. If you do decide to share a taste of these with baby, heating them until steaming can reduce the risk of foodborne illness; just let it cool before offering.

→ **Foods high in mercury.** Certain fish, such as Chilean sea bass, swordfish, and certain varieties of tuna, contain high levels of the heavy metal mercury, and infants are particularly susceptible to its negative effects.

→ **Unpasteurized (raw) dairy.** Since the immune systems of babies and young children are still developing, they can be especially susceptible to foodborne illness from unpasteurized dairy products such as raw milk and raw cheeses.

→ **Raw sprouts.** If you enjoy incorporating bean or vegetable sprouts into meals, cook them thoroughly before offering to baby, or hold off until the child is older, since sprouts can be associated with an increased risk of foodborne illness for babies.

→ **Alcohol.** Many of us have heard that alcohol "burns off" during cooking, but it's a bit more complicated than that. How much alcohol remains in a dish can depend on the type of alcohol used, how the dish is prepared, other ingredients present, cooking time, and more. Babies and young children are more sensitive to the negative impacts of alcohol in food, so, while this might feel abundantly cautious, it's better to be safe and keep alcohol out of food when possible. Make sure to keep alcohol (including cooking alcohol and extracts) out of reach in the kitchen as well, as accidental alcohol ingestion by babies is more common than we realize. Vanilla extract and other similar flavorings are fine when used in small amounts in cooking.

→ **Caffeine.** Avoid drinks made with caffeinated ingredients, like coffee and caffeinated teas, and be mindful of foods with caffeine. An occasional taste is fine, but caffeine should be generally avoided in the diets of babies and young children.

Keep the Kitchen Clean

Life is busy, time gets away from us, and there's always too much to do. When you're prepping food, make your life easier in the long run by taking steps to keep germs and illness at bay. You can help your future self by keeping cooking areas clean, separating foods to prevent germs from spreading, fully cooking dishes, and shortly after cooking, chilling foods in the fridge to reduce the risk of the growth of unfriendly food germs and foodborne illness.

Some Great First Foods

The following foods are terrific options as first foods for babies. For how to safely prepare these foods for baby's age and developmental ability, see our First Foods database in the Solid Starts App.

Fruits and Vegetables

Apple
Asparagus
Avocado
Banana
Beet
Bell pepper
Bok choy
Broccoli
Cabbage
Cantaloupe
Carrot
Celery
Chayote
Corn on the cob
Dragon fruit
Durian
Green beans
Honeydew melon
Kiwi
Kohlrabi
Lotus root
Mango pit

Nopales
Papaya
Peach
Pear
Peas
Persimmon
Pineapple core
Plantain
Plum
Potato
Quince
Sapodilla
Star fruit
Summer squash
Sweet potato
Taro
Tomato
Turnip
Winter squash
Yam
Zapote
Zucchini

Proteins and Fats

Arctic char

Beans

Beef brisket

Burrata

Chicken drumstick

Chicken liver

Cottage cheese

Cream cheese

Duck

Eggs

Flaxseed (linseed)

Fresh goat cheese

Ghee

Goat meat

Ground beef

Ground lamb

Hemp seed

Kefir

Labneh

Lamb rib bone

Lentils

Mascarpone cheese

Mozzarella cheese

Paneer

Peanut butter

Pulled pork

Pumpkin seed butter

Quark

Rainbow trout

Ricotta cheese

Salmon

Sardines

Sour cream

Spare rib bone

Steak

Sunflower seed butter

Swiss cheese

Tahini

Tempeh

Tofu

Tree nut butters

Turkey

Yogurt

Grains and Pseudo Grains

Amaranth seed

Barley

Bread

Buckwheat

Bulgur

Cracked wheat

Fonio

Freekeh

Millet

Oats

Rice and wild rice

Rye

Sorghum

Spelt

Teff

Tortilla

Helping Baby Tolerate Spice

If you eat a lot of spicy food, consider toning down the spice level at first for baby to help them acclimate. We recommend a "low and slow" introduction to spicy foods. Mixing them with other creamy foods such as yogurt, mashed potatoes, or plain rice can take the heat down a notch to keep baby from experiencing any physical pain or digestive discomfort. Incorporating sweet foods with the spicy ones can help, too. You can increase the level of spiciness little by little over time.

How About Drinks?

A 6- to 12-month-old baby's main drinks are breast milk, formula, and a small amount of water (unless directed by baby's medical provider). Avoid cow's milk or milk alternatives, coffee, tea, juices, soda, or any other drink that can displace their intake of breast milk or formula until after 12 months of age. In some countries, cow's milk or an appropriate calcium-fortified milk alternative may be introduced around 9 to 12 months of age. To decide if this is appropriate for your baby, discuss with your baby's medical provider. While small amounts of water (1 to 2 ounces) in a cup each mealtime can be helpful for constipation and to practice cup drinking, it's not a requirement and there is no need to push baby to consume any certain amount. For more information on cup and straw drinking, see Chapter 12. For more information on cow's milk and milk alternatives, see Chapter 15.

Introducing Allergens Early

While it is possible to be allergic to any food, the most common food allergens include cow's milk, egg, finned fish, peanut, sesame, shellfish, soy, tree nuts, and wheat. We'll dive into common food allergens, including best practices for introducing them, in Chapter 14, where you will learn about introductory approaches to suit every style, whether you prefer to take it slow or get right to it.

Iron-Rich Foods

One nutrient to keep in mind as you're planning meals is iron. Around 6 months, baby's iron stores from birth have naturally decreased. While formula in the United States and to a lesser extent breast milk continue to provide iron for babies, iron-rich foods can also help meet baby's iron needs once baby is developmentally ready for them. Around 9+ months of age, many babies are learning how to eat more solids to help support their overall nutrition and iron levels. The goal is to regularly offer iron-rich foods and trust that, with time, practice, and patience, baby will learn the skills to consume the iron and nourishment they need.

Iron is an important nutrient that baby needs to support their development. In industrialized countries such as the United States, rates of iron deficiency in infants and toddlers are estimated to be around 15 to 20 percent, depending on the study, and about a third or more of these infants and toddlers may experience iron deficiency that progresses to iron deficiency anemia—when the red blood cells become smaller and symptoms often become more pronounced.[9,10,11] Symptoms of iron deficiency include, but are not limited to, pale complexion, increased fussiness, low energy, trouble with sleep, decreased appetite, frequent illness, and delayed development. Iron deficiency anemia can occur for a wide variety of reasons: low iron intake from food, increased iron needs due to medical conditions, medication side effects, genetics, and other uncontrollable factors. If you have concerns about baby's iron status, don't hesitate to connect with a pediatric healthcare provider for more support.

Many foods marketed to infants and toddlers don't offer adequate iron and aren't well suited to support the development of their feeding skills either.[12,13] Some families opt for iron-fortified infant cereal as their go-to source of iron, but there are also many other iron-rich and baby-friendly foods already in their kitchen and pantry. We encourage you to begin serving these foods to baby when you start their solids journey.

Iron-Rich Foods (Animal-Based)

Beef	Goat
Bison	Herring
Chicken	Lamb
Duck	Mackerel
Egg	Sardines

Iron-Rich Foods (Vegetarian)

Beans	Oat cereal (iron-fortified)
Chickpeas	Pumpkin seeds
Edamame	Tahini
Kidney beans	Tempeh
Lentils	Tofu

Jars, Puffs, and Pouches

The baby aisle at any grocery store is packed with jarred baby foods, pouches, puffs, baby cookies, baby crackers, and teething biscuits, so let's talk about them for a moment. Contrary to popular belief, there is no obligation to offer these foods to your baby, and it is perfectly fine to skip these if you prefer. These products also keep baby eating different foods from the rest of the family and reduce baby's exposure to flavors that the family enjoys. In addition, they are not as effective as family food at helping baby build important oral motor skills. That said, prepared baby foods can offer families significant convenience as something that can be quickly grabbed and served to baby with little to no preparation. In the case of purees, they are often included in government- or nonprofit-provided food benefits, making them an accessible resource for many families. If you'd like to serve these foods to baby, it is absolutely fine to do so.

Here are a few tips to help weave in these foods while also familiarizing baby with family foods and helping them build oral motor skills when you have the time:

→ Transfer jarred baby food and the contents of any pouches to a bowl for baby to eat with a spoon or their hands most of the time. Babies love to drink directly from pouches and can often figure out how to do so early on because baby is using their sucking skills, not practicing new, more challenging chewing skills.

→ Use purees as dips and spreads for other finger foods from your meal. This allows baby to eat what you eat but also adds flavor and nutrition.

→ Mix purees into sauces, dips, and nut butters.

→ Save puffs, baby crackers, and teething biscuits for times when you are on the go. These foods are just fine on occasion, but many families fall into the habit of serving these at every meal, assuming they are safer than other foods and are teaching chewing skills. These products are considered a "meltable" food, meaning they melt away with minimal chewing, so they do not actually trigger baby's chewing reflexes like other finger foods do. And many babies who often eat these foods quickly develop a strong preference for puffs and teething biscuits, learning early on that they can reject other foods and the parent will present puffs. This can make it challenging to introduce baby to other food flavors and textures during this important time. The solution is to serve these packaged foods in moderation.

Baby's First Tastes of the World

Baby is about to have a wonderful adventure, and you are going to be the one curating this exciting experience for them. Our best advice is to not overthink it. Offer a variety of foods, cooked in the way your family enjoys, including spices and the flavors you love. Choose foods that you want to eat, that are available to you, and that are relevant to you, where you live, and your culture.

Now, as you are starting to let baby practice the mechanics of managing food, is the time to show them the wide range of flavors out there. They're going to have so much fun as they graduate from the sweet milkiness of breast milk and formula to the sweet coolness of watermelon, the warmth of cinnamon, and the savory taste of steak. They'll get a kick out of the various berries and pucker up when they get a hint of lime. And it's going to be fun for you, too—if you've never seen a baby taste a lemon, you're in for an adorable treat.

Summary

✓ Focus on foods that you love when considering first foods for baby. There are many benefits to serving the family meal from the start.

✓ Almost any food can be made safe for babies, which we'll explain in the next chapter.

✓ Explore letting baby eat purees with their fingers or mixing them into other foods.

✓ Have fun, and show baby how much fun the world of eating can be.

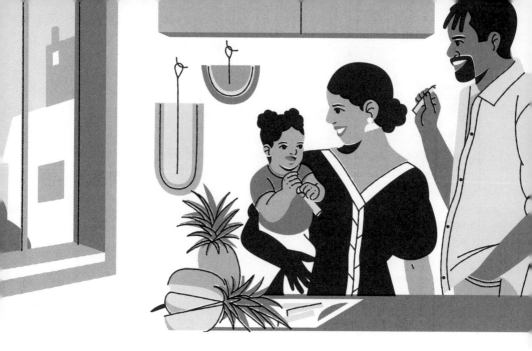

Chapter Ten

Food Prep by Age

One of Maggie's very first foods was pineapple. We had just brought one home from the store and were so excited at how ripe and sweet it was. Maggie was watching us eat it so intently, we had to share some with her. I knew the piece needed to be soft and cut into a stick shape so she could pick it up, and I will never forget the adorable look on her face when she figured out how to get it to her mouth. My husband and I laughed for hours about it!

—Karen, Maggie's mom

E ach food has its own properties and textures. Some are hard and crunchy, some are slippery, some are fibrous, some are chewy. This chapter is a series of lessons on how to prepare all of these various foods for baby depending on the stage of development they are in. Foods properly prepared will help with safety, advancing eating skills, and developing chewing ability, as well as showing baby that yes, you can do it, and yes, there is a delicious payoff when you get that bite into your mouth.

Safety. All of our recommendations for how to cut and prepare food for baby prioritize safety, which means that we prioritize sizes and shapes that can be easily picked up and self-fed by a baby just starting out and minimize the characteristics that are known to increase choking risk.

Advancing eating skills. We want baby to learn to eat what the rest of the family eats, prepared the way the rest of the family eats it. For this reason, we often encourage preparation styles that challenge baby's oral motor skills and build chewing ability. We encourage you to aim to offer a variety of foods with varying textures and flavors.

Developing chewing ability. You might be wondering if it's important to prepare foods in a way to make it easy to get food in baby's belly. We encourage you to try to focus more on exploration and skill development than consumption. As baby builds skills, they will eventually begin eating and swallowing food. If getting food into baby's belly is a priority, there are many ways to prepare foods that increase baby's consumption. Try to balance intake with foods that further baby's chewing skills.

How to Cut and Prepare Food for Baby

Food preparation for baby does not have to be complicated, and with some simple guidance, modifying food (if needed) will become second nature. The primary textures you will introduce to baby over the next several months include the following:

- **soft, scoopable foods,** such as oatmeal or mashed potatoes
- **soft finger foods,** such as banana or peach
- **fibrous foods,** such as strips of cooked meat or asparagus
- **unbreakable foods,** such as meat on the bone or a mango pit
- **crunchy foods,** such as cucumber or bell pepper
- **crumbly foods,** such as a hard-boiled egg yolk or a cracker
- **lumpy, mixed-texture foods,** such as cottage cheese
- **grains and small particle foods** that spread in the mouth, such as quinoa or rice
- **runny foods,** such as soup or yogurt

Soft, Scoopable Foods

While there's no need to mash all of baby's food, soft foods are an important texture to introduce to baby. Many foods that we adults enjoy—porridge, potatoes, or plantains—are cooked until soft and/or mashed until scoopable. This texture is great because babies can often experience success with swallowing the food well before they figure out how to take bites and chew finger foods and move them backward to swallow. Many parents also feel encouraged when they see their child eat and swallow foods, which provides confidence in baby's feeding abilities. It's a wonderful way to introduce common allergens to baby and know that they actually ingested some of it. Soft foods and mashes also provide excellent sensory input and help acclimate baby to more sticky and messy textures as well as runny foods, which can be challenging to convince a toddler (and let's be real—many adults!) to try.

While soft or mashed food may not lend itself to as much chewing development, it can be a way to calm your nerves and feel like starting solids is successful. If this is the case, leave some lumps and soft chunks to get baby used to some texture and aim to add in finger foods by 8 to 9 months. Soft foods are also a great way to practice utensil skills. Foods that naturally coat a spoon are easier for baby to learn to scoop and self-feed.

Here are some soft foods and mashes that cling to the spoon:

Baba ghanoush	Kasha porridge
Bean dip	Mashed avocado
Chia seed pudding	Mashed beans
Congee	Mashed potato
Fufu	Muhamarra
Grits	Oatmeal
Guacamole	Poi
Halim	Polenta
Hummus	Yogurt (thick styles)

Soft Finger Foods

Many foods, like ripe bananas, peaches, and pears, are naturally soft. And soft is also a great texture to aim for when cooking foods for baby: think scrambled egg strips, roasted butternut squash, or tofu strips.

A great guideline for safety is that soft finger foods should be soft enough to mash with a fork or your thumb, but not so soft that they fall apart when baby tries to pick them up. The goal is for the food to start breaking down as baby gnaws or sucks on it. But do know that these soft foods, although easy to mash with the tongue and gums, can cause gagging as they spread on the tongue.

Fibrous Foods

Some firm or fibrous foods, such as a strip of meat or a stalk of as- paragus, can also be great for babies just starting out. These foods hold together well against a baby's emerging jaw strength and tend to cause less gagging. They also provide excellent sensory feedback to baby's tongue and jaw and do a great job of triggering chewing reflexes, so they are exceptional at advancing baby's oral motor skills. They are also excellent for babies who have a more sensitive gag reflex, as they don't spread in the mouth. Although most babies will not be able to fully chew this texture for several more months (meaning most, if not all, of the food will be spit out), these foods are excellent for building skill. If you like, such fibrous foods can be dipped in sauces and purees to increase baby's interest and help baby ingest nourishing foods and nutrients such as iron.

When offered fibrous foods, babies (even new eaters) will occasionally manage to bite off a big piece. While this is expected and normal, it can feel incredibly scary for parents. Trust that baby has all the foundational reflexes to manage that piece and get it safely out of their mouth if needed.

Introduce well-cooked strips of meat and lightly cooked fibrous vegetables, such as steamed broccoli, roasted asparagus, or shredded cabbage, early on. While it may seem safer to wait, these are excellent foods for new eaters to practice with, and getting young babies familiar with this texture early has enormous benefits. Once a baby gets used to eating soft, mashable foods, they sometimes will then refuse more fibrous foods, which require more work to break down in the mouth and can quickly bore baby. Introducing fibrous foods early helps increase the likelihood of baby accepting this texture later on.

Unbreakable Foods

Food teethers are foods that are so firm and resistive that they will not break into pieces in the mouth as baby munches. Some examples include spare ribs with most of the meat cut off, a mango pit, or a pineapple core. As strange as these might sound, these foods are great options for build-

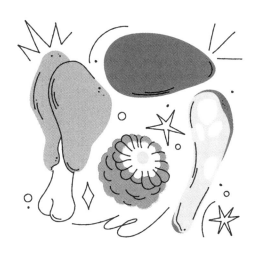

ing baby's jaw control and tongue coordination, and they are unbeatable at helping baby develop the mental map of their mouth (that's the sensory awareness that allows a baby to know where food is in the mouth and if it's broken down enough to comfortably swallow).

These foods stimulate the chewing reflexes, and baby gets repetitive practice moving the tongue and jaw to chew, but the food doesn't break apart in the mouth, so baby does not have to figure out how to move any small pieces around just yet. Because there are no small pieces to manage or bites to be gagged or spit back out, many anxious parents find that unbreakable food teethers are the best next step when moving from purees and mashes to finger foods.

Food teethers are also helpful for babies who have a sensitive gag reflex, and can be a lifeline for babies who get upset quickly when they gag, because unbreakable food teethers can actually help to lessen the gag reflex over time.

> Food teethers can also function in a similar way to a utensil, allowing baby to practice dipping, stirring, and scooping. This is a great way to use purees. Simply put some puree in a bowl and use the food teether to dip in it.

Crunchy Foods

Crunchy foods, like apples, raw carrots, and whole nuts or large pieces of nuts, are a challenge for young eaters and are best avoided in their natural crunchy form at first, since they tend to pose a high risk of choking. However, there are other crunchy foods that can be made safe without cooking them, including cucumbers, "O"-shaped cereals, and thinly sliced bell pepper. To learn how to safely prepare any food for a baby's age and developmental ability, use our First Foods database in the Solid Starts App.

Crumbly Foods

Crumbly foods, like hard-boiled eggs and ground beef, can be challenging for young eaters. They hold their shape until baby munches on them and then they spread in the mouth, which can be hard for new eaters to manage. To minimize the struggle, modify crumbly foods at first. One way to do this is to moisten them. For example, a very soft meatball made with egg and breadcrumbs can help prevent the beef from falling apart into crumbly pieces in baby's mouth. As baby gets better at managing pieces of food in the mouth over time, work up to letting baby experience the crumbly food on its own.

> Foods such as hard-boiled eggs can be mixed with yo-gurt or avocado to moisten them, which helps them cling to utensils and fingers for more successful eating.

Lumpy, Mixed-Texture Foods

Foods such as cottage cheese, guacamole, bean dips, and stews can be excellent first foods to load onto a spoon or to place directly into a bowl for baby to practice scooping with their hands. These foods can expand baby's tolerance to texture and provide a fun sensory experience for baby's hands and mouth. Note that mixed-textured foods often cause a fair amount of gagging as baby gets used to the feeling of the food in the mouth—all the more reason to introduce them early.

Grains and Small Particle Foods

Grains and small particle foods, such as quinoa or rice, are a great texture to try once baby has a bit of experience with lumpy or mixed textures and soft finger foods. Small particle foods can present a challenge for new eaters because they are difficult for babies to pick up and bring to the mouth, and once they are in the mouth, they also tend to scatter, leading to big gags. Moistening these foods with sauce or mashing them with a fork can help bind the grains together—and can make a big difference in baby's tolerance for this important texture. As baby gets better at moving foods around the mouth with the tongue, you can modify them less to help baby learn to manage small-particle foods in the mouth.

Runny Foods

Soups, sauces, dips, and foods such as yogurt can all have a runny texture. These foods provide a wonderful sensory experience for baby and are fun to introduce early in baby's eating journey because often they can be successfully swallowed. You can load them onto a spoon that you hand over to baby, simply serve a small amount smeared on a tray, or place some in a bowl to let baby scoop with their hands. If you have a sensitive baby who tends to gag often with this texture, start by offering tiny tastes of these foods on your clean finger to help build baby's interest in and tolerance for bigger bites down the road.

Safety Modification Guidelines

To minimize choking risk, eliminate or reduce qualities that make food harder for a baby to manage or easier to get lodged in a baby's airway, which is about ¼ inch (6 mm). You'll prepare food in a way that makes it easier for baby to feed themselves, to move food around in the mouth, and to break down the food, which decreases the risk of choking in the rare event of an uncoordinated swallow.

→ **Slippery foods:** If sticky, like avocado, coat in breadcrumbs or infant cereal. If not sticky, like mango, cut with notches to create grip.

→ **Round foods** such as blueberries or grapes: flatten or slice.

→ **Tapered foods** such as strawberries: slice.

→ **Springy foods** such as sausage: slice thinly or shred.

→ **Firm foods** such as apple: cook until soft.

→ **Hard foods** such nuts: finely grind.

→ **Sticky foods** such as nut butter: thin with water.

→ **Rubbery foods** such as shrimp: shred or thinly slice.

It's impossible to eliminate all food risk, and in theory, an individual can choke on any food, but reducing these attributes can make a big impact on baby's safety.

Choking risk is reduced when baby self-feeds the food item. When food is independently picked up and placed in the mouth only by the eater, the risk of choking and aspiration is decreased.[1,2,3,4,5] Foods should always be prepared to allow for coordinated self-feeding based on baby's developmental level.

Common Choking Hazards and How to Modify Them for Safety

This list is hotly debated by healthcare professionals and is somewhat subjective.

As you know, high-risk foods such as hard candies, marshmallows, and gum are worth avoiding altogether. For high-risk foods such as carrots, grapes, fish with bones, and apples, we recommend you modify these foods to make them safer for baby.

→ **Apple:** cook until very soft, or cut into thin slices.
→ **Blueberries:** flatten between your fingers.
→ **Carrots:** cook until very soft, then mash or slice lengthwise; grate raw carrot.
→ **Celery:** slice into thin slivers and cook until soft, then mix into scoopable food.
→ **Cheese:** cut into thin slices.
→ **Cherries:** pit and quarter once pincer grasp develops.
→ **Chickpeas:** smash each one or blend into a mash.
→ **Corn:** avoid loose corn kernels; serve on the cob instead.
→ **Dried fruit:** avoid in dried form; reconstitute in warm water and puree.
→ **Fish:** debone thoroughly.

→ **Grapes:** cook until soft or, once the pincer grasp develops, quarter (lengthwise if oblong).

→ **Melon:** cut into thin slices (never melon balls or cubes) or offer on the rind.

→ **Peas:** smash and mix into a scoopable food such as mashed potatoes, smash once pincer grasp develops.

→ **Pear:** choose a very ripe pear or if it's firm, cook until soft or serve in thin slices.

→ **Nuts and seeds:** finely grind and mix into other foods.

→ **Nut and seed butters:** thin into a loose sauce by mixing with water, applesauce, yogurt, breast milk, or formula.

→ **Oranges, tangerines, mandarins:** remove membrane and any seeds from each segment.

→ **Rice, barley, and other grains:** cook well and mix into a binding food like yogurt.

→ **Sausage:** quarter lengthwise, remove casing if present.

→ **Shrimp:** cut lengthwise into flat halves.

→ **Strawberry:** remove the tapered end and offer whole only if very large and soft; if small and/or firm, smash, slice, or cook.

→ **Tomato (cherry and grape):** avoid at first, and once the pincer grasp develops, cut into quarters.

How We Determine Our "How to Cut" Recommendations

Many recommendations for feeding solid foods to infants lack an evidence base altogether and are influenced by tradition (how it's *always* been done). Others are inconsistent, biased, and incorrect assumptions about safety and skill.[6,7,8] At Solid Starts, we are lucky to have multiple professionals on our team who are experts in not only child development (neuromuscular, motor, and cognitive) but also in development and refinement of oral motor skill. In addition, our feeding and swallowing team has a combined 40+ years of experience in the assessment of normal and abnormal swallowing, from neonates through adolescents and teenagers. Furthermore, our recommendations are reviewed and finely tuned by a double-board-certified pediatrician/gastroenterologist. Put simply, we do not make these recommendations lightly, and we pull from a vast landscape of literature across multiple disciplines. Where we cannot find literature to specifically determine a recommendation, we pull from our clinical experience and knowledge of chewing, swallowing, and dysphagia (disordered swallowing), as well as complementary areas of research such as child development, motor learning, biomechanics, and rehabilitation.

When considering recommendations for how to cut foods to decrease choking risk, we look to:

→ Make it easy for baby to self-feed, given their anticipated fine-motor skills at their given age.
→ Match food to typical oral motor capability and the development of new skills at each age.
→ Keep presentations simple, with the least amount of modifications necessary for safety.

To learn how to safely prepare any food for a baby's age and developmental ability, use our First Foods database in the Solid Starts App.

Preparing Food to Reduce Choking Risk

We know there are seven characteristics that make a food high risk for choking. Our first and most important goal is to identify recommendations that decrease or eliminate those characteristics. For instance, food that is small, round or tapered, firm, compressible, or slippery is more likely to enter and get lodged in the airway and be difficult to expel without assistance, leading to a true choking emergency. We aim to eliminate these factors because baby's safety is our number one priority.

Preparing Food for Self-Feeding Success

Based on what we know about the development of hand skills, infants between 6 and 8 months of age have the coordination to use only the entire hand to pick up an object or rake it into their palm. Therefore, food must be the right size and shape for gross grasping, not small pieces that need to be picked up with the fingertips.

Around 9 months of age, babies develop what is known as a pincer grasp, which allows them to pick up small pieces of food with their fingertips. At this point, babies can be offered bite-size pieces of food because they will be able to self-feed this smaller size.

We'll get into this in greater detail shortly, but for now, keep in mind the following:

→ From 6 to 8 months of age, cut food large at first, so it is easy for baby to grasp.
→ Spears or stick shapes are easy for baby to hold.
→ Adding notches or texture can help baby's fingers keep a grasp on food.
→ Around 9 months of age, consider adding smaller, bite-size pieces of food, about the size of an adult thumb knuckle, to help baby grow their hand skills and chewing ability.

Prepping Food for Baby's Chewing Ability

We know our newest eaters do not have a lot of eating skills yet. They have the reflexes to support building these skills, but the real learning hasn't happened yet. As they learn, we want to keep them as safe as possible, and we want them to be successful but also to stretch toward new skills, fumble, make mistakes, and grow. If we want to advance their skills, we must introduce them to foods that challenge their skills. Don't start with the riskiest foods; start with foods that have been modified to be as safe as possible and then increase the challenge from there.

Imagine coaching a child to catch a ball. Isn't it easier to start with a large beach ball they can wrap both arms around than a small baseball or golf ball that is more difficult to grab hold of? This example applies to food as well. Larger pieces allow baby to use their whole hand to feed themself, are easier for baby to keep hold of and pull back out of the mouth if needed, are better at triggering oral motor chewing reflexes, and are easier for baby's brain to keep track of in the mouth. In time, once they build more coordination, baby will learn to manage smaller pieces.

Food Prep: 6 to 8 Months Old

In general, prepare the food to fit the following characteristics:

- → length and width of two adult fingers
- → or large enough that baby uses two hands to bring it to their mouth

For this age group, stick-shaped foods are generally the easiest for baby to pick up and self-feed, but this is not an essential shape. A large, soft meatball works just as well as a large strip of roasted zucchini. Generally, the bigger the piece of food, the safer it is for a younger eater. The food must be large enough for baby to pick up and feed it to themself, and when baby is holding the food, there should be some sticking out on the top and bottom of their fist.

Babies at this age have reflexes that help them chew and break down food. But an often-overlooked skill required to eat is the tongue's ability to pull those broken-down bits of food back together into a little ball or package that is easily moved to the back of the throat and swallowed. Most 6-month-old babies are going to find that skill very challenging, but if we give them ample opportunity to practice, by serving them soft, mash-able finger foods, most ba-bies will develop this skill by 8 to 10 months of age.

Some 6- to 7-month-olds may find soft, mashable foods challenging because these foods quickly spread around the mouth as they mash or may cling to the roof of the mouth. As the food spreads, it tends to lead to gagging. This is where slightly firmer foods, which start breaking down into smaller pieces with a bit of sucking or gnawing, or highly resistive foods, can also be great options. They allow baby to increase their tolerance to texture and input in their mouth but still enable the control to pull these foods back out of their mouth without leaving mashed food behind.

Making a Mental Map of the Mouth

Research shows that during the 6- to 8-month window, items that provide a lot of touch pressure feedback (also known as "tactile input") to the gums, tongue, and palate along with force feedback (also known as "proprioceptive input") to the jaw and tongue muscles give the brain the most comprehensive and accurate information about what is going on in the mouth.[9] The more tactile and proprioceptive information the brain gets, the more likely the mouth will know what to do with that item.[10] Bigger, firmer pieces of food provide high-value sensory motor learning while also activating the chewing reflexes.

Similarly, the swallow reflex involves a complex series of motor movements, all of which are designed to close off the airway, preventing choking or aspiration from occurring. While swallowing is a reflex, it does its job by getting sensory information from the inside of the mouth and the food. The motor movements of swallowing will change depending on the information the brain gets about the food and how it's moving around.[11]

For example, the duration of time that the airway stays closed when swallowing solid food is longer than the duration of time it stays closed when swallowing your saliva.[12] The mouth collects sensory feedback from the food and passes it to the brain, which quickly sends a message to the throat, telling it what must be done to keep the airway safe during a swallow. The more sensory receptors are triggered by the food, the more information and feedback that food gives the brain and then the throat. Bigger and firmer pieces of food trigger more sensory receptors in baby's tongue, palate, cheeks, and jaw, giving baby's brain valuable information.

But What If Baby Takes a Big Bite?

We'll walk through several common scenarios and questions that parents have when baby first gets started in the next chapter, but this is the question we are asked most often when parents learn that baby can be offered big pieces of food, so we want to answer it before we go any further.

Anxiety around baby taking a big bite of food is normal and expected. While it may appear scary, remember that baby has the reflexes and mechanisms to handle it. When a baby actively takes a bite of a food item, the brain gets the message, "Hey, I'm supposed to chew this." Deep brain stem reflexes are triggered, and baby will most likely engage motor patterns to move the food around in the mouth— spitting it out, swallowing it whole (and yes, this is generally okay!), or possibly gagging on it. You may be tempted to pull the food out, but refrain from putting your fingers in baby's mouth as this can increase the risk of choking by pushing the food back farther into the mouth and toward the throat, taking away baby's control of the food. As tempting as it may be, don't do it.

Spitting Out a Big Bite

1 **Stay calm and be patient.** You don't want to scare baby and, while it may feel like an emergency, it is not. Babies can chew big pieces of food or safely swallow them whole. If they don't spit the food out, try not to assume the worst.

2 **Clear the food from the tray.** Make sure baby does not continue to put more food in their mouth.

3 **Kneel down in front of baby.** As they look down at you, their head tilts forward. This movement puts gravity on your side.

4 **Use gravity if needed.** If baby doesn't lean forward to look down at you, help them by placing a hand on their back and gently leaning them forward.

5 **Talk to baby.** "That's too much. Spit it out." Even if baby doesn't have the language to fully understand your words, talking helps baby associate the word "spit" with the action that you're practicing, and your calm tone helps reassure baby if they're uncomfortable or upset.

6 **Place your hand under baby's chin.** This simple cue, especially when baby is looking down at you, can encourage them to open their mouth and stick out their tongue.

7 **Stick out your own tongue** in an exaggerated way. You can even add a sound effect: "Ahhhh." You can also spit out a small bit of your own food to demonstrate. As you model how to spit, keep your hand under baby's chin as a cue.

Why Don't We Give Small Pieces to Babies?

For the past few decades, persisting even today, many people incorrectly recommend diced and chopped foods for young babies. Diced and chopped foods are too small for most 6- to 8-month-olds to self-feed; these foods require a pincer grasp to successfully bring to the mouth. What babies can successfully pick up are larger strips or chunks of food using an age-appropriate gross grasp (that whole-handed grab we mentioned earlier).

Additionally, young babies can have a harder time managing small pieces of food in their mouth; with that immature map of the mouth and immature tongue control, either those pieces aren't noticed or baby can't figure out how to find them and move them around. If babies do manage to pick up a small, bite-size piece using a raking motion with their whole hand, that piece will get trapped in their fist, as they can't yet move small items from their palm into their fingers.

Food Prep: 9 to 12 Months Old

Around 9 months of age, baby will be improving their gross and fine-motor skills. Of particular importance at this age is the emergence of more refined hand coordination. To date, baby has been grasping toys and food with the palms of the hand. Between 8 and 9 months of age, many babies start to connect the tips of the thumb and pointer finger to form a pincer grasp.[13] Baby's tongue and jaw may also be stronger and more coordinated at tearing foods.

A baby with a pincer grasp can pick up food as small as a piece of cereal, though in time they are eventually able to pick up much smaller pieces, even the size of a grain of rice.

With these skills developing, it's safe to decrease the size of their food. Once baby has the fine-motor skill to grasp a small item and bring it to their mouth, thereby feeding themselves, you can offer them opportunities to explore bite-size pieces. These bite-size pieces can range in size from small to medium (think the size of a postage stamp or adult knuckle), as long as baby can use their fingers to pick them up.

Along with picking up bite-size pieces, around 9 to 12 months of age, baby is developing the skills and ability to self-feed food that is thinly sliced or shredded, such as shredded cheese and meat.

Why Bite-Size at 9 Months?

Around 9 months of age, baby will likely be progressing in their chewing skills, with improvements in tongue coordination and sensory awareness inside their mouth. Your child's oral motor skills have had a decent amount of practice moving around big pieces of food that provide lots of sensory feedback, and they are ready to work on finding and manipulating the smaller pieces.

If baby has been practicing with chewable foods since 6 months of age, by now they also have had a decent amount of experience biting, tearing, and moving big pieces of food. Bite-size pieces are a new challenge and a new step in learning how to eat a wide variety of foods.

Babies at this age commonly overstuff their mouths as they get more confidence in self-feeding, as well as swallow pieces of food whole. If this happens, continue offering bigger pieces of food (larger than could fit in their mouth at once) to help babies learn how to take a bite, learn about their mouth's borders, and draw a "mental map" of what fits and what doesn't.

Food Prep: 12 to 17 Months Old

At 12 months of age, a toddler can likely chew a wide variety of textures and sizes if they have been practicing chewing solid foods for a few months. At this age, a toddler can likely eat what you eat with a few modifications, such as:

→ Cut the food into small pieces (perfect for utensil practice).
→ Provide foods that are soft and large, such as a banana, so the child has to take bites.
→ Provide foods that are sliced or shredded.
→ Cook resistive foods requiring a lot of chewing until soft, or serve in thin slices, shreds, or dice.
→ Continue to thoroughly cook meat, poultry, fish, and eggs.

Toddlers may continue spitting out some foods that aren't chewed well, especially until their molars come in, allowing them to more effectively grind challenging textures; this is normal. If spitting happens, offer stick- or spear-shaped foods to help the child further "map" the mouth and develop more refined chewing skills.

Frequently Asked Questions About Sizes, Shapes, and Textures

If I'm starting finger foods around 9 months of age, do I use the 6-month-old size or bite-size pieces?

The simple answer is you can use either, but we find that starting with exposure to bigger pieces of food can be beneficial. These big pieces of food are easier for a new eater to figure out how to move around and build baseline manipulation skills. If you are starting after the pincer grasp emerges, you can pair both sizes of foods and lean on bigger pieces if baby is having a hard time with the smaller ones. For more help on this transition, check out Chapter 13.

Why go down in size at all?

The easy answer is you don't have to, but it is a good opportunity for baby to learn new skills. In general, going down in size may increase how much baby gets into their belly, but for some babies this isn't the case. These new sizes and shapes are a learning experience for baby. While some babies take the skills they built on chewing bigger pieces of food and immediately apply them to manipulating smaller ones, other babies do a lot of spitting when figuring this out. It's an excellent idea to offer both big and small pieces of food to baby so they can continue to build more gross manipulation skills and improve their biting and tearing, while also refining their skills with smaller pieces.

Why not just give purees at first and then wait until baby is 9 months old, then move directly to small, bite-size pieces?

Put simply, babies need to learn how to move the tongue and jaw around to get those small pieces chewed. Those movements are built with the bigger foods. For many years, parents were taught that babies who are just starting solids should be served only small, bite-size pieces of food, that big pieces of food were a choking risk. This myth persists to this day, though it has no research to support it. If anything, research is more supportive of the building of chewing skills during the period from 6 to 8 months using larger-sized foods.[14,15,16] If you start with small, bite-size pieces of food, baby will not be able to pick these pieces up until closer to 9 to 10 months of age and baby will lose out on months of practice and skill building before the nutrition from solid foods becomes more important. Babies are not inherently safer with chewing at this age if they have not had consistent practice chewing over their first couple of months of starting solids. Remember: research has shown that infants have a developmental window between 6 and 8 months of age for learning to chew, with the most willingness and strongest reflexes to help them learn and keep them safe. If finger foods aren't started until around 9 months of age, baby will miss this window, making it a bit more challenging—not impossible, but harder to learn to chew.[17,18,19]

Summary

✓ From 6 to 8 months, go big. Larger pieces of food are easier for baby to self-feed (which reduces choking risk) and are easier to manage in the mouth.

✓ Around 9 months of age baby will develop a pincer grasp, which will enable them to pick up smaller pieces of food. At this time you can move to bite-size pieces of food if you like.

✓ Explore all the food textures: soft and scoopable, fibrous, hard and unbreakable foods, crumbly, crunchy, lumpy, and runny.

✓ When serving finger foods, be sure to cut them in shapes and sizes that baby can pick up by themselves. Spears or stick shapes are easy for baby to hold, and adding notches or texture can help baby's fingers keep a grasp on food.

✓ Firm, slippery, and small, round foods can be choking risks, so read through the guidelines for serving blueberries, grapes, or cherry tomatoes (and other foods).

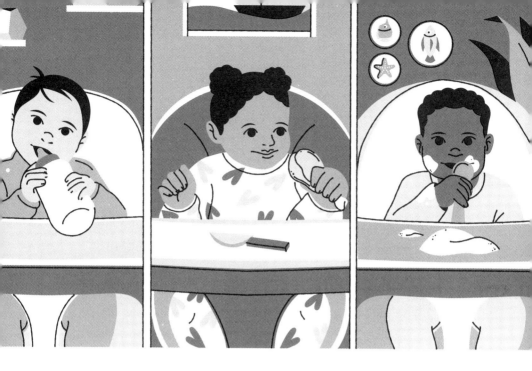

Chapter Eleven

Go Time

Zuri's parents both came from families with strong food cultures, and they were very excited to share their love of food with Zuri. Once she showed signs of readiness for solids, they wanted to jump right in, and they decided to simply start sharing food off their plate so Zuri would be exposed to the flavors of their cuisines right from the beginning. Zuri was up for the challenge. By 9 months, Zuri was eating two meals a day and mostly eating versions of what the rest of the family was having.

Alex's mom came to this stage with some of her own fears. Afraid of offering Alex chewable food, she stuck to just one meal a day of purees and mashes until he was 8 months old. She let him explore purees and mashes with his fingers, enabling him to take the lead with feeding himself. When he was particularly tired or cranky, she skipped the pureed meal. At 8 months, Alex began reaching for food on his mom's plate, so she introduced food teethers like a mango pit and corn on the cob alongside his mashed food. Soon after that, around 9 months, she felt confident enough to offer modified versions of what she was eating, and Alex used the self-feeding skills he had been practicing from the beginning along with his new oral motor skills to build chewing skills, happily joining in on the meal once or twice a day.

Some parents are ready to dive into solids the moment baby is ready ... and some want to get in the pool a little more cautiously. Welcome to the magic window—where baby is ready, and you get to choose the pace.

There are many ways to accomplish the ultimate goal of getting baby eating what the family eats. Some parents, like Zuri's family, move directly to finger foods. Some, like Alex's, choose a more conservative start to solids with a gradual progression from purees and mashes to finger foods. We've used two examples here to show that even in this enriched learning window, parents will have different ideas about how to structure their journey, and kids will have different ways of taking to the task—and that's okay. Choose the pace that feels right for you and matches baby's temperament and communication. While you may want to go slowly or jump right in, baby will likely have their own opinions as well.

When you first start bringing baby to the table for meals, keep the portions small. At first, a meal might look like just one or two pieces of food. You can keep a few more pieces ready on your own plate in the likely event baby wants more.

In this age window of 6 to 8 months, baby is ready to learn how to chew and is likely the most willing to explore new foods than at any other time in their life. The next 2 to 3 months are all about introducing baby to a variety of flavors, textures, colors, sizes, and shapes of food. This will be a big change for them—and for you, too. The amazing thing is that you get to do this in a way that works for you and for baby. Pacing is personal, and babies are quite adaptable, so how you proceed is up to you.

Go time works a bit differently for babies who are blind or have low vision, and for babies who are deaf or hard of hearing. Visit SolidStarts.com to learn more.

Go Time Primer

As you've learned, nearly any food or meal can be made baby-friendly with a few easy tweaks and attunements—no separate meal or short-order cooking required. When you decide to offer baby their first food, keep things easy, manage your expectations, and try to have fun.

You don't need to manage baby's eating. You do need to manage your expectations. Baby may not swallow much or even touch the food at first, but you can trust that with practice and modeling, baby will learn. There's no need for any well-intentioned counting of bites. No need to obsess over nutrition. Even when you really, really, really mean well, research has shown that this mindset can lead to increased pressure and strain baby's relationship with food.[1,2]

The First Few Meals

Start with simple, single-ingredient options for baby's first few meals. Baby does not need a full plate of food but rather a single piece of food, like a bit of fruit or vegetable or a piece of meat or fish from your meal. As for amounts, you'll follow baby's lead, not any strict guidance on serving sizes.

When cooking food you know you'll share with baby, reduce added sugar and salt when you can. When you can't, just share and enjoy the foods you have anyway. The most important thing is building a positive food experience. (We'll go over sugar and salt in Chapter 15.)

The First Few Weeks

You can serve a food again a day after offering it for the first time, or you can move on to other flavors and choices. The old advice was to introduce the same food for three days in a row before moving on to the next. This is not necessary. In fact, it has been shown to hinder the introduction of a wide variety of foods in the first year. Again, it's okay to introduce two or more new foods that are not common allergens at the same time (or over the course of the same day). You will also aim to introduce egg, peanut, and dairy in the first few weeks of solids. See more on allergen introduction in Chapter 14.

What This Might Look Like

In the morning, you might prepare your own breakfast, which could be a bowl of yogurt with granola and a pear. You can put a thick-cut wedge of pear on baby's plate to let them explore, dipped in a bit of yogurt to introduce dairy (a common allergen). Hold off from sharing any granola as it has a lot of nuts and hard clumps in it.

Another day, you may be eating a spiced rice dish with chicken drumsticks. You can offer baby a chicken drumstick with the skin removed. If baby appears to be enjoying the activity, you can then serve some of the spiced rice on top of yogurt to reduce the heat. If baby is excited and engaged, you can offer more.

Portions and Food Waste

In these first few weeks to months, we recommend thinking of meals as exploratory. Let baby play with and explore their food on their own terms. Doing so, however, will inevitably lead to mess and sometimes wasted food that gets squished or falls to the floor.

Food waste is a valid concern because, truthfully, baby won't actually eat much of the food you serve in those early weeks or even the first month or so. This is another reason to keep portions small at the start and to use a splat mat to catch any fallen food.

If the food ends up on the floor by the end of the meal, you'll have lost only a little. And this early investment in exploration, which may feel wasteful at first, can significantly decrease food waste later on. Less bringing home lunchboxes uneaten, less going back to the kitchen to make a second meal because the first was refused, and less buying of special baby foods that won't be eaten by other members of the family.

Every table meal experience builds on the last. Within a few short weeks, you'll have a much better idea of what baby is capable of, what size food seems to work best, and how much food you should bring to the table so that you and baby have the best mealtime possible.

Purees, Mashes, and Spoons

If you are taking a more gradual approach and starting with purees and mashes, keep these things in mind:

- Starting with very small tastes can prepare baby for what's to come. Offer a taste on your finger, or even smear some puree on their tray or table for them to explore.

- Loading spoons can be a great way to let baby take the lead. Dip both ends of the spoon in the puree so they have more opportunities to be successful in case they use the spoon upside down.

- Check out Chapter 9 for some great options of purees and mashes that stick well to a spoon.

- If you want to control the spoon, don't forget about responsive spoon-feeding (see Chapter 5). Hold the spoon out for baby and wait for them to lean in, open their mouth, and accept it.

- Plan to move toward having baby hold the spoon and self-feed earlier rather than later to avoid baby developing a strong sucking pattern in response to food.

Almost Everything Is Normal

When baby first joins you in a meal, they will watch you eat at first, and may begin to copy you. If they're used to seeing people eat, they may try to get the food into their own mouth at once. Or they won't. Both are normal.

Normal baby behaviors with food include the following:

→ Smashing
→ Squishing
→ Dropping
→ Throwing
→ Pouring/dumping
→ Windshield-wiping
→ Banging
→ Grunting
→ Spitting
→ Gagging
→ Biting off big pieces
→ Biting food, then fussing
→ Shuddering
→ Shivering
→ Making funny faces
→ Not eating much
→ Eating a lot one day and not much the next
→ Blowing raspberries

→ Meals taking 5 minutes   → Meals taking 30 minutes

→ Kicking legs   → Pushing to stand up

Try to avoid inserting judgments around whether baby likes or dislikes something based on their immediate expressions. Babies will explore flavors that you might not even dream of putting in your mouth, make a horrified face, then go back for more. So even if they act like they do not like it, avoid saying so. Instead say things such as "You're not sure about that flavor yet" or "That was new for you" or "You're all done with that one for now." You can also say things such as "I see you touched that" or "I know this is all new." If you're not sure what to say, just focus on narrating what you see baby do. This is mostly for you, not baby. Baby might not yet understand the words, but they do understand and will respond to your soothing, supportive tone. It's okay if they don't do anything and you just finish your meal. Many times, less is more.

We want to repeat: even if baby doesn't touch or eat anything, this is still a successful meal. Learning to eat solid food will take time and practice.

Babies Do Not Eat Politely

Babies are born with many useful reflexes. Table manners are not among them. If baby does interact with the food, they will likely squish, squeeze, windshield-wiper, bang, drop, or throw it. All of this is expected and a part of the learning process. While it can be hard, try not to discourage this exploration. You can introduce utensils (more on utensils in Chapter 12), but know utensils are another challenging new skill for baby and it will take months of practice to get it right. While table manners are a goal for many families, know that the cognitive and motor skills needed to politely eat take years to hone.[3]

Mealtime mess engages multiple sensory systems at once: taste, touch, smell, sight, hearing, and body awareness. These sensory experiences allow baby's brain to make an educated guess about how the food will feel and move within their mouth. As baby squeezes an item in their fist, their brain learns more about how much force might be necessary to break apart this food with their jaw. All of these sensory inputs from the food help build connections in baby's brain and encourage the development of motor skills and problem-solving capabilities.[4]

Food-sensory play can increase acceptance of new and varied foods by allowing for baby's brain to get information and feedback about different types of food properties, such as texture, temperature, color, smell, and state (sticky, smooth, hard, soft) and to become comfortable with these properties.[5] Letting baby explore and touch and have different textures on their body decreases the likelihood of baby developing sensory sensitivities to various textures.[6,7,8] Some babies are just naturally less interested in getting messy and do not eagerly dive in to exploring foods. For most babies, this is a normal temperament variation. If this describes your baby, turn to page 300 in the Problem Solving section to learn more.

Avoid the urge to bypass the mess by hand-feeding baby or constantly wiping baby's face. We've discussed the many downsides of overcontrolling behavior from the parent during mealtimes, but frequent cleaning of baby's face and hands can also cause issues. Few babies like to have their face wiped, and most flat-out hate it. If baby associates the high chair with getting wiped down, they may start avoiding sitting in the high chair altogether. Over time, overzealous cleaning can also result in baby not being able to stand mess on their body.

If a Mess Gives You Stress

Some parents are particularly stressed out by the mess created at mealtimes. It's perfectly fine to pick and choose days or times when you feel capable of handling the mess and cleanup and allow baby to self-feed, while you spoon-feed or hand-feed baby at the other meals (if baby will allow this). If the mess is a particular problem for you, offer lots of food teethers—unbreakable sticks of food. These foods, such as corn on the cob and meat on the bone, have the incredible advantage of being the least messy (and are amazing for oral motor skills). Knowing that the mess has immense value can alleviate some of the stress around it and make it easier to tolerate. Other families prefer to keep a damp washcloth at the table and teach baby early to wipe their hands on it periodically. Rather than wiping baby, you can wipe your own hands, then offer baby the cloth to touch and imitate you. Often baby will catch on quickly and begin trying to clean their hands whenever you offer the cloth. Giving this prompt but ultimately allowing baby to have control can be a respectful way to minimize mess.

Frequently Asked Questions About Go Time

A few very common situations come up that parents tend to be concerned about. Here are some common questions:

What if baby doesn't seem interested?

If baby isn't automatically reaching for the spoon or food and bringing it to their mouth, we've got you. Get baby in the high chair and make sure they can reach the table and see you. Poor positioning in the high chair is a common barrier to participation. See more on high chair positioning in Chapter 8.

Once you are certain baby is positioned for success, be sure baby knows what is expected of them. Catch baby's attention by smiling and cooing at them, then bring the food to your own mouth in an exaggerated way. Whether you are using a spoon or a piece of food, place a bite dramatically in your mouth. Show that you are enjoying the eating experience. Say "mmmm" liberally. Chew with your mouth open so baby can see what's going on in there. Do this once or twice, then hand the loaded spoon or piece of food over in the air to baby, which sends the message, "This is for you to hold."

If baby does not imitate you and does not reach out for the food, set it down in front of baby, then keep showing them how much you are enjoying your own food, but pause the show periodically for baby to look around and notice their own food.

During the first meal (or even the first few meals) baby might not do anything but watch you. That's completely fine, and there's no need to change anything. At subsequent meals, be sure to try this again with different sizes, shapes, colors, and textures of food to see if anything seems to capture baby's attention and interest in exploring. No need to try to hand-feed baby or keep trying to hand them food. They will pick it up when they are ready if you follow a routine of showing up at the table together, sharing food, modeling eating and enjoying food, and moving on when baby has lost interest. If it's still not clicking for baby after a few weeks of trying these basic tips, check out our section on food refusal on page 301 in the Problem Solving section.

What if baby spits everything out?
While it may feel frustrating to watch, spitting food is actually a big part of learning to eat. Babies tend to bite and spit for a while before they figure out how to move the food backward to swallow. Some babies figure this out quickly, while others take a few weeks or months of practice before it clicks. As long as baby is showing the ability to move some easy-to-pass foods back to swallow after a month or so of practice (think a puree or mash like yogurt or oatmeal), just let them keep working on the skill.

Here are two things you can do to help baby move through this stage: (1) offer lots of opportunities to explore food teethers and (2) bring baby to the table a bit hungrier by waiting 45 to 60 minutes after breast or bottle feeding before offering solid foods. Food teethers provide lots of opportunities for the tongue to practice the movements it needs to move the food backward to swallow, and coming to the table a bit hungrier helps with motivation to swallow the food.

If baby continues to spit *all* foods, even soft and pureed consistencies, after 2 to 3 months of consistent practice and coming to the table hungry, consider talking to your child's medical provider about an oral motor/ feeding assessment.

Keep in mind that spitting is also an important skill for baby to have— when they are mobile and putting a variety of things in their mouth, having the motor skill to spit unsafe objects is crucial.

What if baby doesn't spit? Coach them!

1 While away from the table, stick out your tongue at baby and pause. Wait for baby to imitate you. You can also try gently tapping their chin as you stick out your tongue.

2 Demonstrate spitting yourself. Exaggerate putting something in your mouth and spitting it into your hand dramatically.

3 Get a clean washcloth, put a corner of it in your mouth, and shake the cloth in front of baby. Wait for them to reach out to touch/grab it and, when they do, let go and laugh. Try again, making a game out of the activity. Each time they pull on the cloth, dramatically say "blah" and stick out your tongue to mimic spitting. Try to play this game where baby puts the cloth in their mouth and you gently pull on it and say "spit out" to get them to open their mouth to release the item.

It can take months of practice for baby to become an expert spitter. Do not give up. With consistent modeling and practice, the child will figure it out.

What if baby coughs?

While coughing is often confused with choking, remember that coughing and choking are not the same thing—and coughing is a sign that air is flowing through the airway. If baby is coughing, let them work it out on their own. Offering a drink of water or putting your fingers in their mouth while they cough tends to make it worse. You can kneel down next to baby so they look at you and remain calm while they cough. This is just a sign that their body is doing the right thing to keep food away from the breathing tube.

What if baby breaks a bigger piece into smaller pieces?

If baby can break apart the food, it is likely soft enough for the gums to munch as well, but the key is if they can get it to their mouth independently. The main tenet of safe feeding and swallowing is self-feeding. If a baby has the skill to pick up a small piece of food (i.e., pincer grasp), it is safe for them to feed it to themself. Most young babies who break food apart do not have this skill and will struggle to pick up small pieces of food, which means they are not able to bring these smaller pieces to their mouth. If you are ever concerned, remove those smaller pieces of food from the tray. For more tips, see page 295 in the Problem Solving section.

What's Up with This Poop?

Once baby actually starts consuming solids, their poop changes. You'll see a difference in consistency, frequency, color, and overall smell. It is very normal to see tomato skins, mushroom pieces, outer shells of corn, bean skins, and other fibrous food pieces that are hard to digest in baby's poop. So long as baby is otherwise thriving, this is nothing to be concerned about. Consistency is more important than number of bowel movements. If bowel movements are soft and easy to pass, pooping every day or every few days can be normal. If they begin to become firmer and drier, consider introducing a few ounces of water per day. Check out the Problem Solving section on page 305 for more tips.

Summary

✓ Choose the pacing that feels right for you and baby.

✓ Choose food that you like, serve some to yourself and some to baby, then eat together.

✓ Some babies take right to eating. Some need more time. Both are normal.

✓ Babies are very messy eaters. The good thing is that this doubles as sensory play.

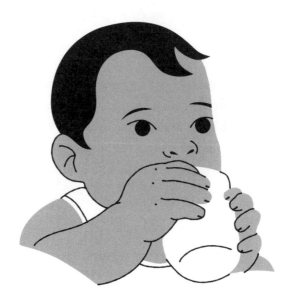

Chapter Twelve

Teaching Cups, Straws, and Utensils

Nicole didn't start introducing cups to Ella until she was almost 8 months old. When they first tried, Ella wanted nothing to do with the cup. But if Nicole just set it down on the table, Ella knocked it over or poured out the liquid. We encouraged Nicole to pause on bringing the cup to the table for a few days and instead hold Ella and walk around with this same cup in her hand (not at mealtimes) and take sips from it. When Ella seemed interested and reached out, Nicole could help her take a small sip of the water. Ella was more interested in letting her mom help with the cup when they were not at the table. After a week, Nicole brought the cup back to the table and Ella picked up the cup and brought it straight to her mouth. She immediately dumped the whole amount on her face, of course, but when Nicole refilled the cup with just a small amount of water, Ella let her mom help control it. After this, Ella was much more interested in the cup at the table and taking drinks from it, which slowly helped her learn to control the cup on her own.

Cups, straws, and utensils can all be introduced around 6 months of age. In fact, we recommend getting started with cups and straws early. Yes, it's one more thing to add to an already busy schedule, but many babies take to cups and straws faster when they are introduced earlier.

Utensils can come later. Using a utensil effectively is a complex fine motor skill that also requires good hand–eye coordination, making utensils a huge challenge for a baby who is still figuring out how to pick things up and keep hold of them. If baby seems interested in utensils because they see you maneuvering your food with those shiny silver tools, bring one to the table to introduce them to the concept. We'll talk more about how to do this in a way that avoids frustration and helps baby learn, and we'll walk you through what you can do to get baby interested in using utensils in toddlerhood.

Most children will be able to use a spoon well by 18 to 24 months of age and a fork by age 3—but it is not at all uncommon to see children continue to use their hands for more challenging-to-hold foods until they are 5 or 6 years old.

Cups and Straws

Introducing cups and straws early capitalizes on baby's desire to explore with their mouth, their strong sucking skills from breast- or bottle-feeding, and their emerging desire to imitate their caregivers. Here's how to do it:

→ Let baby play with cups and straws and get used to having them near or in their mouth.
→ Introduce a cup or a straw each time baby is offered solids.
→ Alternate from meal to meal or from day to day, but it's ideal to practice with both cup and straw during this period.
→ Offer water, breast milk, or formula in baby's cup.
→ Expect this to get messy.

If you are expressing breast milk, you may not want to use it in the beginning as baby learns because much of the contents of the cup will be spilled, and liquid from the straw is probably going to get spit out.

If you choose to practice with water, keep in mind that the American Academy of Pediatrics recommends that infants around 6 months of age can have 4 to 8 ounces of water per day. We tend to err on the lower side, recommending 2 to 4 ounces per day, as water can displace the valuable nutrition from breast milk or formula that baby is drinking.

Remember, learning to drink from a straw and a cup are two new skills for baby to learn. Building skills takes time and practice, so don't be discouraged if baby doesn't get the hang of it right away.

Choosing a Cup

We recommend using a normal open cup instead of a sippy cup. Drinking from an open cup is a lifelong skill, unlike the skills required to drink from a sippy or a spout cup, which will be discarded after a few months or years. There is a hot debate within the feeding therapy and dental communities about whether sippy cups and no-spill, spoutless sippy cups (known as 360 cups) have any negative impact on oral development and oral motor skills. There is currently no convincing evidence to support any negative impacts from any specific type of cup. From our perspective, it's just less work to teach a baby to use the same kind of cup that they will use in childhood. Look for a cup that holds a few ounces or less.

Teaching Baby to Drink from an Open Cup

Cup drinking at this time is simply for practice. Start by pouring in about an ounce of liquid. Baby is learning how to get the cup to their mouth, get the liquid out of the cup and into their mouth, and manage liquid in the mouth differently, so small amounts are better at the beginning. You may hear some coughing at first. This is to be expected and nothing to worry about.

You can hold the cup out for baby to grasp and help them bring it to their mouth, guiding their hands around the cup. Avoid pouring liquid into a baby's open mouth. We want them engaged and trying to drink. You can help baby stabilize the cup on their lower lip and tilt it just enough to bring the liquid into their mouth. You may see baby lap up the liquid or suck it into their mouth; both are okay. Spills are also very common. As baby learns, there will be many mistakes before they get it right.

Some babies resist having things brought to their mouth or simply just want to do it themselves. This is normal. If baby does not like the guidance, allow them to try to do it on their own. Be prepared as it's likely baby will tilt the cup back way too far and pour water all over themselves. When this happens, just coach them: "Oops, too much." You can add a tiny bit more water and let baby try again. If it spills again, no need to refill it this meal. Just set the cup aside and wait until next time.

As baby gets more coordinated, you can start to set the open cup on the table at meals and allow baby to pick it up and drink independently. If baby playfully dumps the contents, do not replace it at that meal and calmly let them know: "Uh-oh, water all gone." Of course, if baby accidentally spilled their cup, use your judgment about offering more. Just avoid starting a game of "I spill my cup and my parent fills it back up."

As with everything, model, model, model. Show them how you drink from your cup, bringing it to your mouth and placing it on your lower lip. Exaggerate holding the water in your mouth and swallowing it. And finally, be patient. This skill isn't easy and takes time for babies to figure out.

Remember, it's not uncommon for this skill to take a while to click, and it's completely normal if baby continues to spill and make mistakes well into early toddlerhood.

Choosing a Straw Cup

Choosing a straw can feel overwhelming. Despite many opinions on when and how to use a straw and what kind, there is no consensus or strong scientific evidence that clearly links the type of straw a child uses to feeding, swallowing, dental, or speech outcomes. What we do know is that your child drinking from a straw, any straw, will help them drink from other straws they may encounter in the future—exposure and practice here are the big takeaways. Ensuring your child is using a clean straw is often more important than the type. That said, here are a few things to think about when choosing a straw:

→ **Diameter:** The narrower the straw, the slower the flow. If your child seems overwhelmed by a standard straw, consider using one that is a little bit narrower. A coffee stirrer can be a great choice.

→ **Material:** While some children may anecdotally do better with one type over another, there is no strong literature to support what material of straw is best, though some manufacturers list product-specific age. There is also concern for hard straws and the danger of toddlers falling with these straws in their mouth.

→ **Length:** If your child is having difficulty sucking liquid up, a straw that is shorter may help.

→ **Valved/Unvalved:** Some straw cups come with valves that keep the cups from leaking if turned over. In order to open the valve, a child needs to bite down on the straw while sucking. In general, we recommend unvalved straws. Valved straws will flow faster if the child bites down, which may encourage a child to bite on any straw they use. But a valved straw is a nonspill option, so if it makes sense for you to use one, just rotate it with a standard straw at other times.

As always, the best way to keep your child safe is to ensure that they are seated and supervised as they learn the skill of straw drinking.

Teaching Baby to Use a Straw

Some babies, especially those close to 6 months of age, just get it on the first try. When offered a straw, they begin to suck, no practice needed, because they are very familiar with sucking from breast- and bottle-feeding, and they figure out how to use that pattern successfully on a straw.

If baby does not immediately catch on to the straw, or if you're introducing the straw to a baby who is a little older, you may need to teach them to close their lips and suck. After modeling (bringing your straw to your mouth and exaggerate kissing lips), there are two main ways to do this.

The pipette method. This method uses a standard straw. Use your finger to trap a small amount of liquid in the straw. Hold the straw relatively vertically out toward baby and wait for them to open their mouth and accept it. Once they close their lips, take your finger off the end of the straw, allowing the liquid to pour into their mouth. Practice this a few times as long as baby is interested. Each time you offer the straw, slowly move it into a more horizontal position so baby has to do a little bit more work to bring the liquid out of the straw. If baby still doesn't get it, no big deal. Put the straw away until the next meal. Usually within a few tries, baby will figure out how to suck the liquid out of the straw.

The straw trainer method. Straw trainer cups are compressible, and when squeezed, they will bring liquid up the straw for baby to drink. These cups introduce baby to the idea that liquid comes up the straw, so they realize they should suck on it, too. Many cups on the market allow you to gently squeeze them, priming the straw, without being marketed as a "straw trainer."

If the pipette method did not work, here's how you can employ a straw trainer cup. Bring a straw trainer filled with water, breast milk, or formula to the table and offer the straw to baby by holding it in front of their mouth. Let baby open their mouth and lean in to accept the straw. Squeeze the barrel a little, which will express a small amount of the liquid into baby's mouth. Most babies will respond by immediately sealing their lips to swallow, which helps them learn to close their lips around the straw.

After practicing like this several times, you can offer the straw trainer to baby, but do not squeeze. Wait and see if they try to get the liquid out on their own by sucking. It may take several introductions, but once they understand how to consistently use the straw and no longer need the squeeze feature, you can transition to other straw cups to generalize the skill to all straws.

If baby does not seem interested in taking the straw in their mouth, that's okay. First, let them spend more time watching you drink from a straw while they play with their straw. You can also dip the straw in a favorite taste, like applesauce or even breast milk or formula, to encourage baby to accept the straw.

Frequently Asked Questions about Cups and Straws

What if baby bites the straw?

Biting the straw is normal because infants are seeking jaw stability. You can exaggerate and demonstrate taking sips from your own straw by opening your mouth wide, then showing your kiss lips on the straw. Some babies will mimic you saying "ahh" after a sip, which can discourage biting.

Practice with the pipette method so you can position the straw on the lips before the teeth, and so baby has an opportunity to gently close their lips and then immediately feel liquid coming out of the straw.

What if baby spits out liquid from the straw or cup?

Spitting during straw and cup drinking is very common, as baby is learning how to move the liquid differently in the mouth. If you do nothing, within a month or so of consistent practice, most babies figure this out and the spitting stops. However, if you do want to try to help baby build those skills a little quicker, here are a few strategies:

1. Cut a regular disposable straw in half to make it shorter, and put it into a small cup, making it more likely that baby will pull up a smaller volume when they drink from the straw.

2. Use a smaller diameter straw such as a coffee straw. These little straws help baby learn to seal their lips tightly, which is an essential piece of swallowing liquids. They also get less liquid each sip.

3. If baby is closer to 1 year old and is still not figuring out this skill, try offering a thicker liquid (smoothie, kefir, etc.)— something that will move more slowly into their mouth so when they pull it from the straw or cup into their mouth, they will have more time to coordinate their swallow. Once they have that feeling down of sucking the liquid up and swallowing, you can return to thinner liquids.

Sometimes a very full open cup helps. With a very full cup, they can suck/slurp at the rim to get the liquid into the mouth, and sucking tends to lead to swallowing.

Some babies figure out that they can purposefully spit out the liquid each time they take a sip. When this happens, try to feign indifference so as to not reinforce the behavior, but also put a quick stop to it by removing the cup. You might say, "Water is for drinking," with a neutral face, then move the cup away from the table for a while. Lean into the behavior away from the table at a time when the behavior is more appropriate. For example, with spitting, you might allow baby a cup of fresh water while they are in the bath to allow them to spit all they want. Or show them how to use this action functionally to rinse their mouth after teeth brushing and spit the water into the sink. Or do so outside. That way you fill their need to explore this fun activity, but you let them know that there are certain spaces where it is appropriate, and certain situations where it is not. When you return to the table, you can remind them that "water is for drinking," and if they keep spitting, you can remove the cup and let them know that there will be time to play with water later.

When can a baby use a cup independently?
While there is a broad age range for when a child will achieve this skill, most toddlers can successfully use a cup between 18 and 24 months of age. Expect occasional small spills even through age 3, which should further improve as your child's graded fine motor control and focus improve. That said, many children can independently use a straw cup much earlier than this, closer to 12 months of age if they started practicing at 6 months of age.

What if baby always coughs when drinking from a straw or cup?
Typically, we see this behavior stopping after a few months of consistent practice. If a baby or toddler is struggling, you can try the same strategies we employ for spitting.

If your child continues to cough when drinking after you employ these strategies for a month or so (or sooner if baby has other unexplained medical concerns such as fevers, frequent upper respiratory infections, or prolonged coughs), bring it up with their medical provider, as a swallowing assessment may be warranted.

What if baby isn't interested in the cup or straw?
If baby does not seem interested in a cup at first, do not pressure them and try to remain neutral about this. Some babies simply aren't interested until they are weaned from bottle- or breastfeeding, and that's okay, too. You can bring empty cups to a play mat outside of mealtimes to build baby's interest. You can add water play by allowing baby to pour from one cup to another or to dip the cup into a larger bowl to scoop the liquid.

Another effective strategy is modeling so baby is motivated to imitate you. Let baby watch you drink from a cup at each meal or between meals. If baby consistently resists, try moving away from the table and holding baby while you drink from a cup, then offering baby a sip. Continue to bring the cup to mealtimes and keep it near baby, ready for them should they change their mind, and know that very likely they will reach out and give it a try at some point.

> Ana, Julian's mom, introduced both a straw cup and an open cup at the table starting around 7 months. She would sometimes bring a small open cup to the table; other days she would bring a straw cup. Julian just played with the straw cup at first, but when Ana used the pipette method to show him that liquid could come out of the straw, he seemed much more interested in it. She then put the straw back in the cup and added a tiny smear of applesauce to the straw to entice Julian to close his lips around it. When he did, she gave the cup a little squeeze, which pushed some water into his mouth. He looked surprised, then went back for more.

After that, it "clicked" for him. Julian preferred a straw cup, and by 8 months he was taking about an ounce of expressed breast milk from the cup during solid food meals.

Fingers or Utensils? Let Baby Choose

We generally suggest letting baby choose whether to eat with their fingers or utensils rather than enforcing one or the other. Many babies figure out that eating with their fingers is faster (using utensils is hard for them!) and will ignore spoons and forks for a while. Don't forget, most kids will figure out how to consistently use utensils somewhere between 18 months of age and the third birthday, so don't expect a lot in the beginning. Babies pick up utensil skills by mimicking what the adults around them are doing, so if you just want to let baby figure it out on their own, you absolutely can.

Model

Demonstrate how you dip a spoon into the food, then scoop, pierce, or stir the spoon around to coat it. Show baby how you bring it to your mouth. Every time baby watches you complete a skill, their mirror neurons are firing, laying the groundwork for doing the same skills themself. No need to bring utensils to every meal, but having spoons or forks occasionally available for practice can help.

Preload Spoons and Forks

When it comes to spoons, start by preloading thick, easy-to-scoop foods like Greek yogurt or labneh, smashed avocado, or even whipped cream. Dip the spoon and either hand it over to baby or place it in front of them so they can pick it up on their own. Consider dipping both ends of the spoon into the food so that baby will be successful regardless of which end they put in their mouth. You can also pre-poke a piece of food on a fork. Some babies respond well to a funny sound like "Boink!" when you poke the food. It's okay if the wrong end goes in their mouth or if the food ends up falling off. Mistakes lead to learning. We also love using big, deep spoons such as measuring spoons to improve a toddler's efficiency in scooping.

Frequently Asked Questions About Utensils

What if baby won't hold or grab the spoon?

If baby isn't interested in grabbing the spoon or wants you to hold it, it's okay to do so, but slow your pace and be sure to pause between bites to feed yourself your own food. This provides modeling and allows space for baby to change their mind and reach out on their own when they are ready. You can also hold the spoon a bit farther away than baby is used to, to encourage them to reach for it.

What if baby frequently drops the spoon?

This is completely normal. You can replace the spoon whenever baby drops it, or you can remove it and allow them to continue eating with their fingers or scooping with their hands, without the distraction of the spoon. Simply try again with the spoon at the next meal.

What if baby just plays with the spoon?

If the spoon becomes a distraction, it's okay to remove it and let baby eat with their hands for a few days before trying again. Or bring the spoon to some meals and not others. In time, as baby builds coordination and more interest in the food, they will likely start using the spoon as a utensil instead of a toy.

What if baby dumps or plays with their plate, bowl, or placemat?

This is normal and expected as baby learns that they can pick these items up and that it's fun to watch the food fall to the floor. If the plate, bowl, or placemat becomes a distraction, remove it from mealtimes for the next few weeks and serve the food directly on the table. For more on what to do with throwing food, see the Problem Solving section on page 295.

What if baby (or a young toddler) refuses to use utensils or is really struggling?

Utensil skills are complex fine motor skills that take time to hone. If baby or toddler is not interested or is really struggling, play with utensils away from the table. Practice scooping dry goods or water in the bath; use a fork to poke play dough. Using utensils during playtime can be a great way to introduce them to a hesitant baby.

Summary

✓ Start cups and straws early. It's easier to teach when babies are young and certain reflexes are in play.

✓ A straw is one new skill; a cup is another. It may take a while for baby to build both of these new skills, so keep your patience around during these learning sessions.

✓ Utensils can come later, unless baby shows eagerness to mimic your utensil use.

✓ You can let baby choose whether to eat with their fingers or utensils. Eating with their fingers is faster, so they may ignore those spoons for a while. Most kids will get the hang of using utensils between ages 18 months and 3 years.

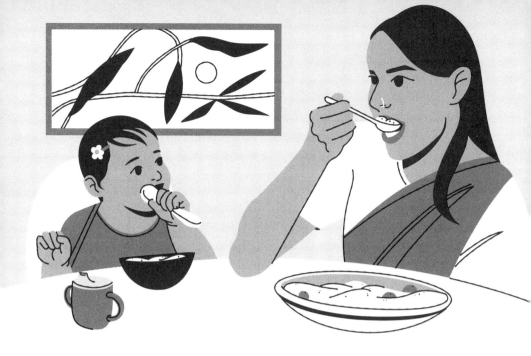

Chapter Thirteen

Spoon-Feeding to Self-Feeding

Mariella had been spoon-feeding her 10-month-old, Leo, purees since they started solids at 5 months of age. When he wouldn't take purees anymore, she knew it was time to give him real food, but, in her words, the thought of doing so "keeps me up at night thinking about him choking and dying." Mariella didn't know how to start, and she wasn't sure how to get over her fear. She reached out to us to help her find her way forward.

f baby is 8 months or older and has been primarily fed purees or mashes, it's time to transition to finger foods and self-feeding. For some babies, this transition is easy and they naturally begin picking up food and bringing it to their mouth with little effort. Other babies need a bit more guidance. As you move from purees to finger foods, know that this is a new skill, and learning new skills takes time and focus.

As you introduce chewable foods and let baby feed themselves, you might see a decrease in the amount of food actually swallowed at each meal. This is normal as baby learns the new skills. If you are worried about how much baby is eating, we recommend offering more formula or breast milk during this transition (rather than relying on more purees to fill the belly) to support this new learning.

How to Begin

Remove distractions, such as toys, from the table. You might even remove plates, bowls, cups, and placemats from the table for a few weeks if these are distracting to baby. Reduce conversation for a few days and keep language brief and straightforward. Simplify your language like "You try" instead of "Okay, now it's your turn and you can try it!" or "Put here" instead of "This is where your spoon goes." Use pointing, body language, and props to show baby as you tell them.

Ideally, baby is calm, happy, and able to focus, and giving them a bottle or a nursing session 45 minutes to an hour before they come to the table is the way to go. Remember, this initial period of transitioning from spoon-feeding to self-feeding is all about exploration and skill building, not consumption at first. Use formula or breast milk as a safety net to meet their current nutrition needs as they learn, so even if they swallow no solids, the meal is still a success. Move on and offer a nursing session or bottle 45 minutes or so after if you think baby is still hungry or has eaten very little. As baby gets the hang of eating solid food, you can slowly move away from breast and bottle feeds shortly before and after mealtime. This way, baby has a bit more hunger drive to eat solid food to fill their belly.

A Gradual Approach

If you'd like to move at a slower pace, pair chewable foods with purees. One way to do this is to serve the same food two ways so baby has a choice. For example, you might serve a mango spear along with mango puree, or an avocado half next to mashed avocado. You can also use sticks of food as the utensils to eat the purees, like a mango spear that baby can dip in yogurt or a cooked vegetable stick to dip in hummus. If you'd like to offer purees and finger foods separately, we recommend starting with a small amount of spoon-feeding to prevent baby from becoming overly hungry and frustrated (but not enough to fill baby up), and then offering time for baby to explore finger food.

Slowly Decrease Purees

Some families choose to start with finger food and then top off with purees, but a word of caution here: babies learn very quickly that eating chewable food is much harder than sucking puree off a spoon. It's common to see babies avoid the chewable food altogether, waiting for the spoon/purees to come out. This makes weaning off purees a bit more challenging. Over time, you want to slowly decrease the amount of pureed food you offer as baby gets the hang of self-feeding and chewing.

Self-Feeding with a Spoon

We generally recommend letting baby learn to feed themselves with their fingers at first. But if baby has been introduced to solids through purees and is use to being fed by the parent with a spoon, they can benefit from learning to self-feed from a spoon first. Since learning to chew and manage finger foods is another layer of challenge, sticking with mashes and purees a bit longer might be beneficial for your child.

Don't be discouraged if baby makes a big mess, misses their mouth, or spills the food all over. This is a normal part of the learning process.

> Leo was very used to being fed but was also beginning to refuse the spoon. We started off by helping Mariella provide Leo opportunities to feed himself with the spoon. He readily reached for and grabbed the spoon without any pressure. Mariella was so proud.

Here are some tips on supporting baby in self-feeding with a spoon:

→ Use spoons that are easy to hold and "grip" the food, and have a few extra spoons available at the table in case one falls.

→ Use foods that are easy for baby to scoop and practice successfully filling the spoon. Foods such as Greek yogurt or mashed avocado can be great to start with.

→ Model loading a spoon and then taking a bite while baby watches. Then load the spoon again and leave it in front of baby; if they don't grab it, make sure they see it. Capture baby's attention by tapping the spoon or saying "here."

→ Hold spoons vertically in the air, just in front of baby. If you need to, you can hold the spoon out for baby to lean in with their mouth and slowly back away every couple of bites to encourage them to reach with their hands.

→ If baby still does not try to reach for the spoon, pick up the spoon and tap baby's arm or hand while holding the spoon out to them. If this is not enough, try placing the spoon into their hand. If needed, try to guide their arm or hand toward the spoon from behind by guiding them by the elbow gently (you could even do this standing behind them). If you feel any resistance from baby at all, stop, as you don't want any hint of "forcing."

→ Teach baby how to dip and scoop by modeling how it is done. After baby takes a bite, put the spoon on the table instead of back in the bowl. Point to the bowl and say, "You do." If they don't try to dip, you can help them dip the spoon again. Be gentle and social as you offer support. Some parents will load up a second spoon and then hand that one over so baby drops the first spoon, but we want baby to learn to keep holding on to their spoon and dip again, so we would use this strategy sparingly.

→ Eat with baby, modeling what to do. This keeps your hands busy, so baby has more of a chance to jump in and do it themself.

→ Build scooping skills away from the table if needed before expecting these skills at mealtime. Here are three ways to do this:
  • Practice digging in the garden with a shovel.
  • Move dirt from one bucket to another with a spoon.
  • Add spoons to water play in the bathtub or outside.

Keep in mind that being fed is easier for baby than feeding themself. As suggested previously, you may want to try to spoon-feed a few bites before tasking baby with feeding themself. This allows them to not be super hungry when they need to do the harder work of feeding themself and sends a signal that it's "mealtime." Some babies will self-feed for a few bites and then want to be fed, and that's okay too, as long as you slowly work to increase the amount of time they self-feed versus you feeding them.

Finger Foods

Start with Unbreakable Food Teethers

Unbreakable food teethers are the easiest way to build chewing skills. These foods are exciting to see (big, bright), easy for a baby to pick up and move in and out of the mouth, and trigger the reflexes that lead to chewing. Food teethers also help baby figure out that sucking to swallow won't work for chewable foods—they need to move the tongue differently to successfully eat these foods.

Follow Up with Softer Finger Foods—and Go BIG

After a week or so, move on to softer finger foods, and we suggest you go big in size (see food preparation suggestions for 6 to 8 months of age in Chapter 10). These larger pieces tend to be easier for a baby just learning to chew. Bigger pieces are easier to bring to the mouth, easier to remove from the mouth if needed, and easier for the brain to recognize and move around the mouth. These bigger pieces continue to develop their new chewing skills before you move down to smaller sizes that require more coordination. Smaller pieces tend to be easier to move around after having experience with bigger ones.

Bite-Size Pieces for Babies with a Pincer Grasp

If baby has a pincer grasp, it's also safe to start with the smaller, bite-size pieces (the 9-month+ serving suggestions). If you're noticing that baby is trying to swallow these pieces whole, gagging, or struggling a lot with smaller pieces of food, going big can help the brain get a better understanding of food in the mouth.

Although she was feeling much more comfortable, Mariella was still nervous about giving Leo finger foods. After he got the hang of feeding himself with the spoon, she started using unbreakable food teethers as dippers and let Leo eat mashes off things like a mango pit. Leo loved munching on food teethers, and this decreased Mariella's stress level as she saw how much he could do. After a month or so of practice, she began to feel comfortable offering bite-size pieces of food, and Leo was enjoying all of the new foods.

Show Baby What to Do by Doing It Yourself

No matter which path you choose, the single most important thing you can do to help baby transition from spoons to fingers is to eat with them, sharing similar or the same foods so that you can model all the skills you want baby to learn. Often pulling their chair right up to the table helps with this. Some babies need to sit on their parent's lap right at first. Capture their attention, be dramatic but slow, and repeat as many times as needed. Give baby a chance to imitate you. It may feel silly, but babies learn by watching us.

Summary

✓ If baby is 8 months old and primarily eating purees or mashes, transition to finger food and self-feeding now. The earlier you start, the easier the transition will be.

✓ Some babies will take to finger food seamlessly. Some need more guidance as it requires new skills, and learning new skills takes time and focus.

✓ We generally recommend letting baby practice feeding themself with their fingers (not utensils) at first.

✓ If baby is use to being fed purees by the parent with a spoon, they can benefit from learning to self-feed from a spoon first.

✓ Modeling helps here. Eat with baby and show them what to do.

✓ Baby is going to make a mess on the way to learning, and that is to be expected.

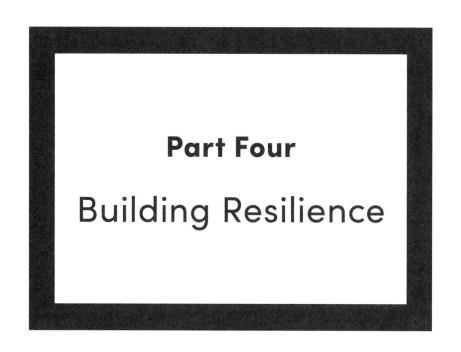

Part Four

Building Resilience

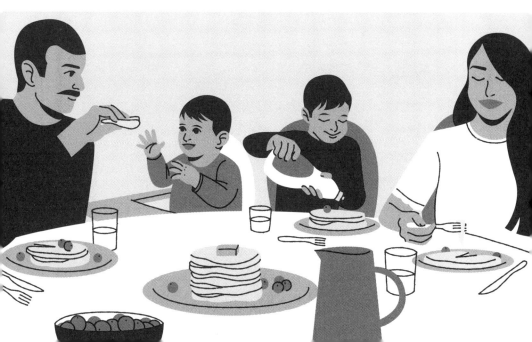

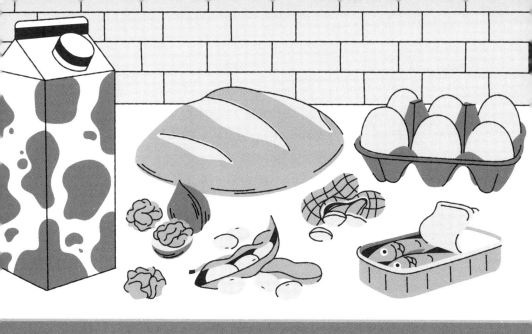

Chapter Fourteen

When (and How) to Introduce Allergens

My 6-month-old baby, Tavi, started solids recently, and mostly he just plays with his food. My doctor told me that I should introduce peanut as soon as possible, and I'm so nervous. What do I do if he has an allergic reaction? And will it even count if he's not swallowing much food yet? Wouldn't it be better to wait until he's older?

—Meesha

Families of children with food allergies are constantly alert, working hard to protect their kids from the risks of accidental food allergen exposure. While most children with food allergies will never experience a life-threatening reaction and will be able to enjoy a wide variety of foods safely, this is primarily due to the diligence of their families. Food allergy families know how much effort that safety takes and what a strain it can be.

This is exactly why we are so focused on getting the message out to parents of infants that the risk of developing food allergies can be reduced with a proactive approach to allergen introduction. Food allergies have been on the rise in recent decades, and increased awareness of the condition has put food allergy front and center in any discussion about solids introduction. It seems that everyone knows someone whose child has experienced an allergic reaction. So Meesha's concerns are totally understandable. However, most babies won't experience any food allergies at all. We have said this before, and we will say it again. Most babies can introduce common food allergens without any issues, but delaying introduction may actually increase the risk.

> You can take steps to reduce a child's risk of developing food allergies, and the biggest one is this: introduce common allergens early.

When it comes to the majority of food allergies worldwide, there are a handful of foods that are usually responsible.[1] Technically, it is possible to be allergic to any food, but when an allergy pops up, the culprit is usually on this short list of common food allergens, which includes eggs, milk, peanuts, tree nuts, soy, seafood, sesame, and wheat.

It's understandable to be nervous about introducing a potential allergen to a young baby who is just learning to eat. We're here to make the case for early introduction of these common food allergens for some important reasons.

One is that introducing food allergens early can actually prevent food allergies. There is strong evidence demonstrating that early introduction of (and regular exposure to) a common food allergen can help prevent an allergy to that food from developing, especially in babies who may be at increased risk. What an opportunity! Simple steps taken early in baby's solid foods journey may prevent them from developing food allergies altogether, protecting them from food, health, and life stresses down the road.

Another strong reason not to delay allergen introduction is that a controlled, gradual exposure to food allergens can result in a milder reaction than if an allergic reaction were to occur outside the home in an uncontrolled setting (such as at school or daycare, at a friend's house, or while traveling) where an unknown amount of the food has been offered. When you introduce allergens intentionally, you have more control over what foods are offered, in what quantities, and under which circumstances.

Additionally, there is immense value in knowing about an allergy as soon as possible so you can take immediate steps to meet with a doctor, learn how to recognize and treat allergic reactions, make a plan with baby's caregivers, and adjust baby's diet to avoid accidental exposure to known allergens in the future.

Finally, the sooner you know about a food allergy, the sooner you can take steps to pursue treatments that may help the child, such as immunotherapy, which can help reduce the severity of symptoms (and in some cases speed up resolution of the allergy). Studies suggest that young immune systems respond particularly well to food allergy treatments, so the earlier, the better.[2]

For these reasons, we agree with Tavi's doctor and encourage families to safely introduce common food allergens as soon as baby is ready, alongside other solid foods. In this chapter, we'll demystify how allergen introduction for babies works and walk you through the steps that you need to take before you get started. We'll also explain how to introduce common food allergens step-by-step.

What Is a Food Allergy?

A food allergy is when the body's immune system mistakenly over-reacts to a food that it should be ignoring. This hypersensitivity can lead to symptoms of an allergic reaction developing quickly (usually within minutes, but occasionally a few hours) after eating that food. Symptoms of food allergy include itching, inflamed rashes (which may look pink or red on babies with lighter skin tones, and purplish or brown on babies with darker skin), drooling, swelling, trouble breathing, vomiting/diarrhea, or a sudden change in behavior or mental status (suddenly very fussy/clingy or sleepy/lethargic). While most allergic reactions to foods are mild and resolve quickly, some reactions can be severe. We discuss how to recognize and treat allergic reactions in more detail in this chapter.

If you suspect that your child has experienced an allergic reaction to a food, stop serving that food and reach out to your doctor. If baby is confirmed to have a food allergy, you will be trained by baby's medical provider to recognize and treat reactions with emergency medication (most importantly, epinephrine for serious reactions), and you should make a plan to monitor the allergy over time, as many food allergies are naturally outgrown during childhood.

What We've Learned

Let's review the science. Although most children will *never* experience an allergic reaction to food, food allergies are relatively common, and some reactions can be life-threatening. In the United States today, 1 in 13 children has a food allergy, and more than 40 percent of them are allergic to more than one food.[3]

Food allergies were noted to be on the rise in the 1990s and early 2000s. In the United States, food allergies in children rose an astounding 50 percent from 1997 to 2011.[4] Interestingly, this is roughly the same period of time during which many parents were advised to wait on introducing common food allergens until well beyond a child's first birthday. In Australia, North America, and the United Kingdom, the feeding advice typically went something like this: No milk until age 1. No egg until age 2. No nuts until age 3. In an effort to protect babies from allergic reactions, they were shielded from food allergen exposure altogether. However, rates of allergy continued to rise. Meanwhile in Africa and Asia, babies were regularly offered common food allergens, such as peanut, as a part of their routine diet. In regions where babies were regularly exposed to peanut, peanut allergy rates remained quite low. Despite the best intentions of doctors in many industrialized nations, their approach to allergen introduction wasn't working.

So you can imagine the shock waves that rippled through the medical community when a 2008 observational study comparing children in Israel and the United Kingdom revealed what some allergists, pediatricians, and epidemiologists had been suspecting: the Israeli infants (who were routinely fed peanut-containing snacks in infancy as a finger food) had a rate of peanut allergy that was *one tenth* that of British infants of a similar Ashkenazi Jewish background who had been advised to avoid peanut exposure.[5] Follow-up research confirmed that the old advice to avoid food allergens was indeed counterproductive. The research is summarized here:

→ In 2015, a landmark study commonly called "LEAP" (Learning Early About Peanut Allergy) demonstrated that the early introduction of peanut to babies at increased risk of developing peanut allergy could reduce the risk of developing the allergy by 81 percent.[6]

→ A follow-up study (LEAP-On), published in 2016, demonstrated that early and regular ingestion of peanuts through age 5 protected the children from developing a peanut allergy later in life, even after a full year of avoiding peanut.[7]

→ Also in 2016, the "EAT" (Enquiring About Tolerance) study provided additional evidence that the early and continued ingestion of a variety of food allergens (particularly egg and peanut) beginning at 3 months of age may prevent food allergies in a general population of young children.[8]

→ In 2017, the PETIT study found that introduction of heated egg (from 6 to 12 months of age) to infants at high risk of allergy due to eczema resulted in approximately a 79 percent reduction in the development of egg allergy compared to egg avoidance.[9]

In response to this mounting evidence, the U.S. National Institute of Allergy and Infectious Diseases changed its recommendations in 2017 to support the early and sustained introduction of food allergens.[10] A 2021 consensus statement from North American allergy societies endorsed these recommendations and emphasized the importance of introducing both egg and peanut to all babies beginning at 6 months of age (as early as 4 months in higher-risk babies) and not delaying the introduction of other common food allergens once solids are introduced.[11]

This approach to food allergy prevention has been supported by expert panels around the world, including the Australasian Society of Clinical Immunology and Allergy (2016), the Asia Pacific Academy of Pediatric Allergy, Respirology, & Immunology (2018), the Canadian Pediatric Society (2018), the Japanese Pediatric Guidelines for Food Allergy (2019), and the European Academy of Allergy and Clinical Immunology (2020).[12,13,14,15,16]

This updated guidance appears to be making a difference: a large Australian population-based study revealed a 16 percent reduction in peanut allergy associated with a threefold increase in the rates of early peanut introduction after implementation of early peanut introduction guidelines in 2016.[17]

Common Food Allergens

The following allergens are responsible for most allergic reactions to food around the world. When planning allergen introduction, prioritize these foods—especially the dietary staples such as peanut, egg, and milk, for which the strongest evidence exists to support the benefits of early introduction. Once these have been introduced, you can proceed with the other common food allergens, as long as eating them aligns with your own family's dietary culture and preferences.

→ Cow's milk
→ Finned fish
→ Hen's egg
→ Peanut
→ Sesame
→ Shellfish (e.g., crab, crawfish, lobster, shrimp)
→ Soy
→ Tree nuts (e.g., almond, cashew, hazelnut, walnut)
→ Wheat

 A Word on Coconut

Even though coconut is a fruit and coconut allergy is rare, the U.S. Food & Drug Administration (FDA) classifies coconut as a tree nut, which means it must be labeled as an allergen by law. In other words, while coconut is not a commonly observed food allergen in the United States, the government requires it to be labeled as such. The FDA acknowledges that their tree nut list is broad and may even contain species with no current food use, but they have erred on the side of having the allergen list be overly inclusive in hopes of protecting those with food allergies.

Understanding Baby's Risk Factors

Some babies are at an increased risk of developing a food allergy. If baby is at an increased risk, it's especially important to take advantage of the protective benefits of early allergen introduction, because these techniques seem to be even more effective in babies at high risk of food allergies. However, depending on the risk factors present and baby's age, you may need to work closely with a pediatrician or allergist before introducing common food allergens at home.

So how do you know if baby is at high risk for food allergy? There are two major risk factors that signal that baby may be more prone to developing a food allergy and therefore may benefit from allergen introduction as early as 4 months of age:

→ eczema, especially severe cases
→ existing food allergy

Read on for a detailed description of each risk factor, but know that if baby does not experience either of these conditions, they are considered low risk.

> If baby does not have an increased risk of food allergy, introducing food allergens at home is a low-risk activity and can be pursued without any special precautions.

On the other hand, if baby experiences one or both of these major risk factors, consult your healthcare team to create a tailored plan to safely introduce potentially allergenic food into baby's diet, order allergy testing (if needed), or supervise early allergen introduction in the clinic.

Family History of Allergy

It is commonly assumed that family history of food allergies is another major risk factor for baby developing a food allergy, but
this is a misconception. There is no strong evidence that the child
or younger sibling of an individual with a food allergy has a significantly increased risk of developing that food allergy themself.[18,19] So you shouldn't assume that your baby will share any
allergies you may have. Allergy specialists now recommend food
allergen introduction at home without any prescreening for babies with a family history of food allergy as long as the child does
not have significant eczema or another preexisting food allergy.[20]
In fact, the deliberate delay of food allergen introduction may
actually increase the risk of the baby developing a food allergy,
especially in cases where eczema is present.[21]

Eczema

Eczema, and severe eczema in particular, is widely considered to be the
most significant risk factor for developing food allergies. (Although
there is no official international definition, most physicians consider
eczema to be severe when the rash covers a large percentage of the
body or lasts for an extended period of time despite regular application
of moisturizers and topical anti-inflammatory medications.)

Up to 20 percent of infants have eczema (also known as "atopic
dermatitis"), an itchy rash that usually appears between 2 and
6 months of age.[22] Eczema is caused by a defect in the skin that allows
moisture and lipids to leave through the outer layer of skin and opens
the door for allergens, irritants, and infections to enter, resulting in
dry, rough, inflamed, and itchy patches. In babies, these patches are
commonly found on the areas that baby can reach to scratch or rub
against, like the face, trunk, and arms or legs. Parents might notice

baby persistently rubbing or scratching these areas, which could lead to skin cracking, bleeding, and possible infection if not quickly addressed. The skin may also develop a thickened texture over time, a result of chronic inflammation. The itching associated with severe eczema can make babies very uncomfortable and irritable, which can interfere with their sleep and feeding.

Although eczema is more likely to occur in individuals with a family or personal history of allergies, experts agree that eczema is not the result of any specific allergy. Rather, eczema increases the risk of developing allergies, as babies with eczema may become reactive to allergens through their outer layer of skin, and the risk increases with time (more time means more exposure to the food allergen through the sensitive skin).

Babies with eczema require special skin care to help heal the skin barrier. Moisturize baby's skin with fragrance-free ointments and creams (which are more effective than lotions), keep baby cool and comfortable, keep nails short to prevent skin damage from scratching, and consult with a pediatrician, allergist, or dermatologist for appropriate medical interventions, such as topical anti-inflammatory medications (which may be needed for moderate to severe eczema).

The most up-to-date food allergy prevention guidelines highlight the importance of introducing common food allergens, such as peanut, into the diets of babies with severe eczema as early as 4 months of age, with the hopes of safely getting high-risk allergens into the diet before food allergy has had an opportunity to develop.[23] Although mild to moderate eczema is associated with a smaller increase in the risk of developing a food allergy than severe eczema, recent studies suggest that all babies with eczema can benefit from introducing peanut beginning at around 4 months of age.[24] In fact, the combined risk of severe eczema with delayed food allergen introduction is high enough that in babies older than 6 months of age, some experts suggest considering allergy testing prior to allergen introduction at home.[25] That said, most medical professionals agree that well-controlled eczema of lower severity does not warrant any special evaluation or testing prior to food allergen introduction in the home setting.

Existing Food Allergies

Babies who already have a confirmed or suspected allergy to one food have a higher risk of developing an allergy to other foods.[26] As we mentioned earlier, 40 percent of children with food allergy are allergic to more than one food. A 2010 study established that babies with confirmed or likely egg or milk allergy were at a significantly increased risk of developing peanut allergy.[27] A decade later, additional studies confirmed that not only egg and milk but other existing or suspected food allergies also contributed to an increased risk of developing peanut allergy in infancy. Allergists have used this data to theorize that the factors that contribute to allergy development for one food simultaneously increase the risk of developing allergy to others as well.

Because of the increased risk of additional food allergies, allergists frequently take a proactive approach to introducing food allergens for these babies, as delaying introduction may increase the risk of additional food allergies developing. However, they may first suggest allergy testing for selected food allergens. Allergy testing measures for IgE antibodies that are specific for particular allergens. IgE is the allergic antibody produced by your white blood cells that recognizes and attaches to allergenic structures on foods. When IgE that is bound to food allergens attaches to the IgE receptor on the surface of the white blood cells in your tissues (skin, respiratory tract, gut, and more), this triggers the rapid release of multiple molecules from the white blood cells, leading to the symptoms we commonly associate with allergy. IgE-mediated sensitization to foods can be tested for with both skin prick testing and blood testing. A negative skin or blood test for IgE to a food allergen suggests that offering that food at home is likely safe. A positive result for a food that has never been consumed can be an indication of potential allergy, but a positive result doesn't guarantee that the food allergy exists and does not mean a food should be automatically eliminated. More than anything, a child's response to eating a food is the gold standard of diagnosis. A positive test result simply means that additional care must be taken to monitor for signs of allergy, and the safest course of action may be to introduce the food allergen under medical supervision in the clinic.

What Can You Do If an Allergy Evaluation Isn't Possible?

Allergy is a fairly small medical specialty, and there unfortunately aren't enough appointments with specialists available to accommodate all the babies who need care. What can you do if baby has severe eczema or a suspected food allergy and you aren't sure how to proceed with food allergen introduction?

1. **Start early.** The greatest risk for food allergy development in high-risk infants is in babies older than 6 months of age. By beginning food allergen introduction (especially for egg and peanut) at 4 months of age, you can take advantage of a window of opportunity to cautiously introduce the allergen at home. (While self-feeding is not practical at this age, babies too young for solids can be offered mashed egg or thinned peanut butter on the tip of a small spoon or clean finger, for example.) If any signs of allergy develop, though, stop feeding and contact your doctor right away.

2. **Work with your pediatrician.** If your high-risk baby is already older than 6 months, your doctor may be able to order focused allergy testing (for just a few relevant foods) via bloodwork. If the testing is negative, food introduction can proceed at home and can open the door to continuing with additional food allergen introduction with greater confidence.

If testing is positive, your doctor may be able to speed up getting an appointment with an allergy specialist because of the time-sensitive nature of the request. Alternatively, in some cases, they may be able to supervise allergen introduction in their own clinic.

3. **Consider a telehealth appointment.** Consider a telemedicine consultation with an allergy specialist who may be able to take a detailed history and offer guidance virtually. Such visits can be a practical approach for families who live far from allergy clinics.

How to Assess Baby's Food Allergy Risk

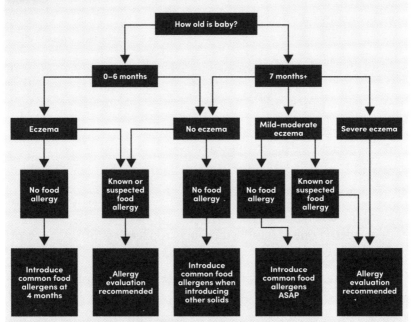

Most babies can introduce common food allergens alongside other foods once they are developmentally ready for solids. However, some babies at increased risk of food allergy may benefit from even earlier introduction or from an allergy assessment before introduction.

How to Spot an Allergic Reaction

The majority of children will never experience an allergic reaction to food, which is a reassuring statistic. However, since up to 8 percent of children may have a food allergy, knowing how to recognize an allergic reaction quickly is important for all caregivers. When reactions are mild, it may not be immediately obvious that your child has experienced an allergic reaction. For example, a baby with egg allergy may develop a single episode of vomiting 15 to 20 minutes after eating scrambled egg. However, when allergic reactions are severe, the dramatic symptoms of the allergy can be unmistakable. An example is a baby who develops eye swelling and repetitive coughing almost immediately after ingesting peanut butter.

Generally, the severity of a reaction is judged by how many symptoms are present as well as their intensity. A mild allergic reaction can include one of the following symptoms (more than one symptom would constitute a more severe reaction):

Symptoms of a Mild Allergic Reaction

→ Itchy or runny nose, sneezing
→ Itchy mouth
→ A few isolated hives, mild itching
→ Mild nausea, gastrointestinal discomfort, or a single episode of vomiting

If you detect one of these symptoms, stop feeding the suspect food and contact your pediatrician, family practitioner, or allergist for guidance. Your doctor may recommend a dose of a fast-acting antihistamine or may advise observation at home or in their clinic.

If the child is showing multiple symptoms at once, however, a more serious reaction may be occurring. Call emergency services immediately and request an ambulance with epinephrine on board.

Symptoms of a Severe Allergic Reaction

Severe allergic reactions (called "anaphylaxis") may include any of the following symptoms, either alone or in combination:

→ Shortness of breath, wheezing, stridor (a harsh, high-pitched noise upon breathing in), or repetitive cough

→ Pale or bluish skin

→ Swelling of face, lips, or tongue (this can result in excessive drooling)

→ Widespread hives on body

→ Repetitive vomiting and/or diarrhea

→ Sudden change in demeanor or alertness, tiredness, lethargy, or seeming limp

If a child shows any of these symptoms, call emergency services immediately and request an ambulance with epinephrine. Do not wait. Allergic reactions can progress rapidly, and epinephrine is the only medication proven to quickly reverse the symptoms of anaphylaxis.

Visit SolidStarts.com for images that show what mild and severe allergic reactions look like on babies of different skin tones.

Do I Need to Keep Allergy Medication at Home?

It is a good idea to keep a bottle of a long-acting, nonsedating liquid antihistamine (like cetirizine [Zyrtec] or levocetirizine [Xyzal]) in your medicine cabinet for use in the event of mild allergy symptoms. These newer antihistamines are better choices than the old standby, diphenhydramine (Benadryl), which has fallen out of favor with allergy specialists because of its tendency to cause sleepiness and its short duration of action.

If your child doesn't have any known food allergies, you don't need to have an epinephrine device on hand "just in case." Most babies won't ever develop a food allergy reaction, so you're unlikely to need it. Additionally, epinephrine devices are expensive and can expire quickly, so they are costly to replace. Finally, shortages of epinephrine devices are not uncommon—so babies who depend on access to this medication can have difficulty getting it if many people without urgent need are purchasing the devices instead.

How do I tell the difference between a rash from acidic foods and an allergic reaction?

If the rash is widespread (such as all over the torso), it is more likely to be an allergic reaction and you should seek immediate medical guidance. Contact rashes from acidic foods (such as lemon, orange, pineapple, and tomato) usually show up in a limited area where baby's skin came in contact with food, such as the chin. Contact rashes typically dissipate within 10 minutes of a gentle cleanse, and there tend to be no other symptoms.

Rashes that occur after touching or eating food may also be associated with hives and itching. This type of rash may or may not go away on its own, and persistent rashes may require medication or medical attention. If the rash does not resolve quickly after gentle cleansing, call your doctor for guidance. There is a chance that the reaction might become more serious if left untreated.

Types of Food Allergies

Some allergic responses are immediate. Some are delayed. And some symptoms that develop after eating food may not be an allergy at all.

It can be confusing to tease out the differences, so let's go over the symptoms of various types of food sensitivities.

Immediate-Response Food Allergy (IgE-Mediated)

IgE-mediated allergy is the classic presentation of food allergy—what we typically think of when discussing an individual who has a peanut allergy and needs to carry an epinephrine device, for example. This type of allergy develops when the immune system produces the IgE antibody that recognizes and triggers reactions to foods that the body should be ignoring as harmless. This is also the type of food allergy on which most research has been conducted and the food allergy that has been shown to be prevented with early allergen introduction.

Timing: A reaction occurs rapidly (usually within minutes, but occasionally a few hours) after eating food.

Common Symptoms: Swelling, red/purplish rashes, itching, respiratory and gastrointestinal distress, low blood pressure (which can lead to poor circulation and neurologic changes)

If a child has an immediate-response allergic reaction to a food, avoid offering that food again until you can make a plan with your doctor. Do not offer the food again on your own, as even a small amount can trigger a serious reaction, and allergic reactions can be unpredictable in terms of their severity. In other words, future exposures may result in a more serious reaction even if the first reaction was not severe. Allergy testing with skin prick tests or blood tests can help to confirm the presence of suspected IgE-mediated allergy. Your doctor can then prescribe emergency medications for you to have on hand in the event of another allergic reaction. The good news? Many food allergies that develop during infancy are outgrown during early childhood, and new treatments are being developed to treat persistent food allergies as well. If available in your area, a visit with a pediatric food allergy specialist can be very helpful as you learn to navigate IgE-mediated food allergy management.

Delayed-Response Food Allergy (Non-IgE-Mediated)

Although not as common as IgE-mediated allergies, other types of food allergies do exist, and awareness of these delayed allergies is increasing. Non-IgE-mediated food allergies generally present with delayed gastrointestinal symptoms, such as reflux, vomiting, and diarrhea. The key difference between IgE-mediated food allergy and non-IgE-mediated food allergy is time: some non-IgE-mediated food allergies may not appear until hours after eating the food, and others become apparent only after the food has been in the diet consistently for weeks or months.

FPIES

Food protein-induced enterocolitis syndrome (FPIES) is one example of non-IgE-mediated (also known as delayed or cell-mediated) food allergy. FPIES is an increasingly recognized food allergy in children, which can be severe and life-threatening in some cases. The classic (acute) presentation of FPIES is an infant who recently switched from breast milk to formula or solid foods. Baby typically begins vomiting between 2 and 4 hours after eating and experiences diarrhea between 5 and 10 hours after eating. Left untreated, reactions can result in significant dehydration. Acute FPIES is extremely rare in infants who are exclusively fed with breast milk.[28] Reactions to FPIES trigger foods can also be chronic and occur when the trigger food is in baby's diet regularly. With chronic FPIES, infants experience frequent vomiting and diarrhea, look unwell, and have difficulty gaining weight. Unfortunately, there are no standardized or validated tests to identify FPIES food triggers, so diagnosing FPIES relies mainly on a patient's history of reactions. Treatment involves avoidance of the food trigger and administration of antinausea medications, IV fluids, and/or steroids for significant reactions. Luckily, most babies with FPIES will eventually outgrow the allergy.

Timing: Typically, a reaction begins a few hours after eating the food.

Common Symptoms: Low body temperature, extreme pallor, and repetitive vomiting and diarrhea, which can lead to significant dehydration and low blood pressure and mental status changes

Food Intolerances

Food intolerance or sensitivity occurs when the body has difficulty digesting a food. This generally results in temporary digestive symptoms that can be uncomfortable, such as gas, bloating, and diarrhea. Although the symptoms may overlap with some allergy symptoms, allergy testing will be negative. Luckily, food intolerances are generally uncommon in babies. If baby does seem to have an issue with a food, a trial of short-term avoidance of the trigger food is reasonable, but keep in mind that many babies experience changes in digestion as their digestive systems shift from taking in breast milk and formula to solid foods. Temporary intolerances, like gas and bloating (such as with beans and broccoli), are normal and expected. In most cases, there's no need to fully eliminate the food, and by offering these foods in smaller amounts and gradually increasing amounts per baby's tolerance, we can set baby up to eat a variety of different foods in the long term. Food intolerances can vary from child to child and can often be dependent on factors like recent illness, antibiotic exposure, gut microbiome adaptations, and more.

Lactose intolerance is an example of a food intolerance that is not a cow's-milk allergy. Lactose intolerance occurs when the body has a hard time processing the lactose sugar that is naturally present in

198 | Solid Starts for Babies

milk. Individuals with lactose intolerance may experience temporary and harmless bloating, gas, diarrhea, nausea, or other discomfort. The good news is that lactose intolerance is uncommon in babies, toddlers, and young children. However, intolerance tends to become more prevalent as children grow older and may affect close to 70 percent of the world's population.[29] For children with lactose intolerance, many lactose-free dairy foods are available. That said, remember that lactose-free dairy products are not safe for children with cow's-milk allergy, as they still contain the whey and casein proteins that cause the allergic reaction.

What Is CMPA?

Cow's-milk protein allergy (CMPA) is not a specific medical term but rather includes both IgE-mediated and non-IgE-mediated cow's-milk allergy.

CMPA is thought to occur in 2 to 3 percent of infants in the United States and approximately 0.5 percent of breastfed babies. Research shows that the majority of children with cow's-milk allergy will outgrow it by age 6.[30]

Many babies with milder symptoms of non-IgE-mediated milk protein allergy (which can show up as painless blood in the bowel movements and is also termed "food protein-induced allergic proctitis," or FPIAP) are able to successfully reintroduce cow's milk before their first birthday, with the guidance of their doctors.[31] Babies with this type of non-IgE-mediated milk sensitivity may also react to soy, but there is not enough evidence to suggest they are at increased risk of developing IgE-mediated allergies to other common food allergens, such as egg or nuts.

How to Introduce and Incorporate Common Allergens

In the next few pages, we'll walk through how to safely introduce a variety of common food allergens. Before you begin, it is important to assess baby's risk factors for food allergy and familiarize yourself with the symptoms of allergic reactions. If you haven't already, please refer to the self-assessment on page 191 and review the guidance on recognizing allergic reactions before reading on.

Tips for Allergen Introduction

While it is important to introduce food allergens early on, we encourage you to start solids with foods that are not common allergens. Once baby has gotten the hang of exploring solids, you can begin introducing food allergens with less worry about normal reactions to new tastes and textures that may be misinterpreted as an allergic reaction. See Chapter 9 for a list of great first foods. If your baby is at high risk of food allergy and is beginning allergen exposures as early as 4 months of age, it is important to follow your healthcare provider's guidance.

Avoid Introducing Allergens on Sick Days

When introducing a potentially allergenic food, offer it on a day when baby is healthy and free of illness. This way, you can pinpoint any symptoms of an allergic reaction to food rather than sickness. By the same token, don't introduce new food allergens shortly after receiving routine childhood vaccines; while vaccination is *not* associated with an increase in development of food allergy, many babies can be fussy or develop a fever after immunization. This can cloud the picture when food allergens are introduced.

Start with a Small Amount

The smaller the quantity of food allergen in baby's food, the less severe the allergic reaction may be. See the allergen introduction schedules later in this chapter for suggested measurements.

Begin in the Morning

When you introduce an allergen in the morning, you have the full day to observe baby, and you are more likely to easily reach your doctor if the child has an allergic reaction. In our opinion, the best time to introduce an allergen is shortly after waking in the morning or right after a morning nap.

Most IgE-mediated allergic reactions occur within minutes of eating the food but can present up to two hours later.[32] For this reason, it is best to introduce allergens at a time when at least one adult can focus their full attention on the baby for at least two hours after eating and avoid distraction from other children or activities. If both parents are working, afternoons or weekends may be better for you. Take your family's individual needs into account.

Introduce One Allergen at a Time

While foods that aren't common allergens can be introduced together, don't introduce multiple common food allergens at the same time—otherwise you will have difficulty identifying the culprit in the unlikely event that a reaction does occur. Pick a common food allergen to introduce and offer it with food that is not a common allergen and that baby has already tried a few times. This way if there is a reaction, you'll know which food was responsible. For instance, if a few days of egg are well tolerated, you can then also add peanut for two to three days, and then begin introducing solid food containing cow's milk. There is no need to trade allergens out for each other—the goal is to continually add more foods to baby's diet.

Consider Baby's Skin

If baby has eczema or sensitive skin, apply a barrier ointment, such as pure petroleum jelly or a plant-based oil/wax combination, to baby's face and hands before mealtime to minimize contact reactions. This helps to reduce the possibility of a harmless contact rash, and it can also help lessen the severity of a reaction if baby does happen to be allergic to the food. Be sure to gently clean baby's face, hands, and skin after the meal, ideally away from the table.

Repeat, Repeat, Repeat

Once you've safely introduced a food allergen to a child, keep that food in the diet routinely. The key to maintaining tolerance is a commitment to regular allergen exposure. Keep each common food allergen in the diet a few times a week if possible (once weekly at minimum). They can be incorporated as ingredients in the meals you prepare. This can look like serving porridge made with cow's milk, wheat flour pancakes with a drizzle of peanut butter or tahini, or egg strips for snacking. Don't stress about the quantity consumed, or if multiple exposures don't occur each and every week, but do try to get each allergen on the menu at least once a week, at minimum. The goal is to consistently maintain food allergens in the diet through baby's fifth birthday, which helps lay a strong foundation for lifelong tolerance.

Don't Rotate Food Allergens

Having lengthy gaps between exposures can defeat the purpose of early introduction. Instead, keep serving them. Continuity counts here.

Grant Yourself Grace

Don't worry too much about volume. If your baby doesn't consume the entire serving of allergen offered that day, that's okay. Relatively modest quantities of allergen exposure (~2 grams or less than two teaspoons per week) can be effective for allergy prevention, as long as exposure remains consistent.

Pick Your Pace

When it comes time to introduce an allergen, some like to dive in while others prefer to take their time. As long as you proactively introduce food allergens, feel free to choose any approach that works for you:

Option 1: Get Right to It. The full portion of the potentially allergenic food is introduced during one meal.

Option 2: Day-Long Introduction. The portion is spread out over multiple meals in a day.

Option 3: Slow and Steady. Portions start small and gradually increase over the course of a few days.

These are all great ways to go about it. One is no better than the other, and these approaches work for every food on the list of common food allergens.

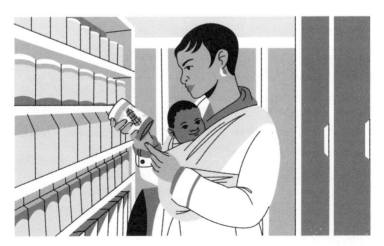

A Step-by-Step Guide

Option 1: Get Right to It

You can introduce baby to a common food allergen over the course of a single meal.

1 Measure 1 tsp (5 mL) of the food allergen you'd like to introduce, such as yogurt; mashed, boiled, or scrambled egg (well cooked, not runny); thinned-out peanut or tree nut butter; wheat farina porridge; thinned-out tahini; or finely chopped and fully cooked fish or shellfish.

2 Dip your fingertip or the tip of a spoon in the food, then let baby taste. Encourage baby to munch on other food while you watch closely. If there is no reaction after 10 minutes, let baby have another taste.

3 Slowly offer the remainder of the food to baby at their natural feeding pace—but only if the child shows interest. It is okay if baby does not want to eat any more today or if they don't finish the full serving. You can try again tomorrow.

Using peanut butter, tree nut butter, or sesame paste (tahini) as an example:

1 Mix together 2 tsp (10 mL) smooth nut butter (honey-free) or tahini with an equal amount of warm water. Set aside approximately half the mixture for today's meal.

2 Dip your fingertip or the tip of a spoon in the mixture, then let baby taste. Let baby munch on other food while you watch closely. If there is no reaction after 10 minutes, let baby have another taste.

3 Slowly offer the remainder of the food to baby at their natural feeding pace—but only if the child shows interest. It is okay if baby does not want to eat any more today. You can try again tomorrow.

Option 2: Day-Long Introduction

You can introduce baby to a common food allergen over the course of one day. Using yogurt as an example (the same approach can be used for many other common allergens):

Breakfast: ⅛ tsp plain yogurt mixed into porridge

Snack: ½ tsp (2.5 mL) plain yogurt alongside fruit or vegetable spears

Lunch: 1 tsp (5 mL) plain yogurt mashed with potato and rice

Snack: 2 tsp (10 mL) plain yogurt alongside fruit or vegetable spears

Option 3: Slow and Steady

You can introduce baby to a common food allergen over the course of three days. Using hard-boiled or fully scrambled eggs as an example (the same approach can be used for many other common allergens):

Day 1: ¼ tsp mashed well-cooked egg alongside fruit or vegetable spears

Day 2: ½ tsp (2.5 mL) mashed well-cooked egg alongside fruit or vegetable spears

Day 3: 1 tsp (5 mL) mashed well-cooked egg mashed with beans

How to Prepare Common Food Allergens for Baby

Some tips on how to prep and serve these important foods:

- **Peanuts:** Thin a teaspoon of smooth peanut butter or peanut powder with water, breast milk, or formula. Ensure that the mixture is well diluted to avoid choking risk from sticky nut butter.

- **Tree Nuts:** Introduce tree nuts through smooth nut butters or finely ground nuts, blended into baby's food. Ensure that the texture is smooth and easy to swallow.
- **Milk:** Start with yogurt or incorporate cow's milk into baby's cereal.
- **Eggs:** Introduce well-cooked eggs, either scrambled or boiled and mashed finely. You can also offer thin strips of an egg omelet as finger food.
- **Wheat:** Introduce wheat with infant wheat cereal or bread-crumbs with minimal added ingredients (no sesame or other common food allergens). As baby grows, offer small pieces of toasted bread or soft, bite-size pieces of pasta once baby is able to pick up these smaller pieces with their fingers.
- **Soy:** Offer soft, mashed tofu in meals or introduce boiled and mashed edamame.
- **Finned Fish:** Start with boneless, low-mercury, well-cooked fish varieties, ensuring that they are mashed for easy swallowing.
- **Shellfish:** Introduce well-cooked shellfish like shrimp, finely chopped or made into baby-friendly patties.
- **Sesame:** Introduce sesame through tahini paste, blended into foods baby is already familiar with.

Remember, all babies can benefit from early allergen introduction, regardless of whether they are at high risk of developing food allergies. However, if your baby is a little older and you haven't introduced allergens yet, don't stress. It's not too late! You can still utilize the approaches discussed above. Refer to the chart on page 191 for guidance on how to assess baby's risk.

Early Introduction for High-Risk Babies

For babies who are at high risk of food allergy, introducing a food allergen may be advised as early as 4 months of age. While this may seem counterintuitive since baby may not yet be ready for solid food, there is emerging evidence that exposure to food allergens at this stage of life can help reduce the risk of developing food allergies. While most babies are not developmentally ready to start solids well before 6 months of age, there are developmentally appropriate ways to introduce common food allergens (keep reading!). For more on developmental readiness for starting solids, see Chapter 7.

For Babies with Eczema of Any Severity

Data from research studies including more than two thousand infants revealed that waiting until 6 months of age to introduce peanut for babies with eczema would miss a critical window of opportunity to introduce peanut prior to the development of the allergy.[33] The longer a baby has eczema, the more likely it is that they will develop sensitivity to peanut through the skin and develop an allergy. Introducing food allergens before that happens can make a big difference.

If your pediatrician or allergist has recommended that baby be exposed to specific allergens at 4 months of age, here are our tips to keep this experience positive and safe from a feeding perspective:

1. Have baby sit on your lap, snuggled in with their back against your belly. This position supports baby's entire body, head, and neck to allow for baby to focus on the task at hand, not holding their body up.

2 Let baby control the experience. Either hold the spoon or your finger out in front of baby and let them visually inspect it first. Let them lean in, open their mouth, and accept the taste. Do not push the food into their mouth.

3 You can also dip a spoon into the food, coating both ends, and hand it over to baby. The food may or may not make it to their mouth, and that's okay.

4 If you have been instructed to expose baby to nut butters, keep in mind that nut butters straight out of the jar are a choking hazard as they are thick and sticky. Thin the nut butter with a small amount of breast milk, formula, or water before offering it to baby to decrease the risk of choking.

Most importantly, follow baby's lead. If baby is not actively engaged, keeps turning their head, or pushes the spoon or food away, consider this behavior as communication that they aren't interested and stop. Watching for cues and respecting them will continue to reinforce trust and connection between caregiver and baby.

What If Your Child Develops a Food Allergy?

Despite our best efforts regarding risk management and allergy prevention, some babies will still develop food allergies. If this is your situation, know that it's not your fault.

It's okay to sit with that initial fear and disappointment when you get the news. Then it's time to roll up your sleeves. Your child depends on you to stay safe and to model resilience and positivity in the face of challenges. You can't change what has already occurred, but you can choose how to manage what life throws your way.

The most important thing you can do to protect your child with food allergies is educate yourself on how to quickly recognize and respond to signs that an allergic reaction is occurring. Review the signs and symptoms of allergic reactions, have a written food allergy action plan from your doctor on how to address any symptoms that may arise in the event of accidental food allergen exposure, and have emergency medication accessible in all the locations where it might be needed (medicine cabinet at home, diaper bag for outings, at daycare or with a babysitter, and even at grandparents' house). Finally, practice using your epinephrine training devices multiple times a year so you are comfortable with the process if the need arises.

Want some good news? Many food allergies, including egg, milk, soy, and wheat, are frequently outgrown during childhood. Additionally, a large percentage of babies with egg and milk allergies can tolerate extensively heated forms of these food allergens in baked goods, pancakes, or noodles, for example. Work with your healthcare team to discuss the best way to monitor the status of your child's food allergy over time. This can include repeat testing via skin test, blood test, or medically supervised oral food challenge. Even for food allergies that tend to be lifelong (peanut, tree nuts, sesame, and seafood), a small subset of patients outgrow the allergy. So never say never!

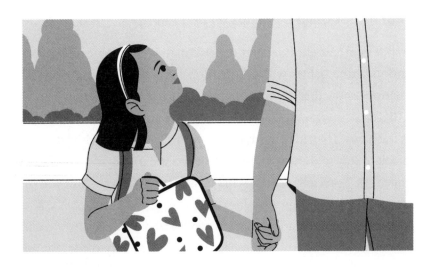

Hope for the Future

As parents, caregivers, and allies to those with food allergies, we are uplifted to know that the field of allergy treatments is constantly evolving. While avoiding known allergens remains the primary strategy for many, we now have treatments available to improve both safety and quality of life for patients with persistent food allergy.

Food Allergen Desensitization

Food allergen desensitization (also known as immunotherapy) is a treatment that uses small amounts of incrementally increasing food allergen exposure to retrain the immune system to gradually become less reactive to the food allergen. In sublingual immunotherapy (SLIT), low doses of allergen are administered under the tongue in the form of liquid drops. In oral immunotherapy (OIT), higher doses of allergen are administered by mouth and ingested. Both therapies can enable patients to tolerate foods labeled for cross-contamination and also accidentally eating a small amount of the food. OIT can, in some cases, allow patients to start eating the former food allergen routinely in their day-to-day diet. There is now emerging evidence that when started in babies and preschool-aged toddlers, these therapies may result in long-term tolerance to the allergen. That said, both treatments require the patient to be exposed to their allergen daily, which is associated with a small (but real) risk of causing a serious allergic reaction. For this reason, food allergen desensitization must only be pursued under the supervision of a certified allergist with extensive experience in the management of food allergy.

Biologic Therapies

Biologic medicines are a class of drugs that are developed using a living system and target specific parts of the immune system to treat disease. Omalizumab (Xolair) is an injectable medication approved for the treatment of IgE-mediated food allergy in individuals 12 months of age and older. When given regularly, it can significantly increase a patient's tolerance for their food allergen and protect them against reactions due to accidental exposure. As time goes on, we expect that additional biologic medications may become available to treat food allergy, giving patients even more options for treatment.

Other Upcoming Treatments

Even for patients who choose to continue actively avoiding their food allergens, new options for the treatment of allergic reactions have recently become available or are on the horizon. These include nasal sprays and under-the-tongue films as alternatives to intramuscular injections of epinephrine for severe allergic reactions. As the fear of an epinephrine injection is one of the major causes of anxiety for families and children living with food allergy, these new options for treatment of allergic reactions have the potential to improve outcomes and quality of life for children with food allergy.

Summary

✓ Introducing food allergens early can prevent food allergies. Once a developmentally ready baby has been introduced to solids, common food allergens can also be introduced.

✓ It's possible to be allergic to any food, but a few are responsible for most food allergies. Peanuts, eggs, and milk are among these common allergens and should be introduced early and then regularly.

✓ Baby is at higher risk of food allergy if they have eczema or an existing food allergy.

✓ If baby does NOT have severe eczema or pre-existing food allergy, common allergens can be introduced in the home setting.

✓ Some babies who are at a high risk of developing food allergy can benefit from allergen introduction as early as 4 months of age.

✓ Introduce one common food allergen at a time. Start small. Build up the quantity of the allergen incrementally over time.

✓ Once introduced, offer common allergens at least once per week (ideally twice per week) throughout the toddler years.

✓ If baby does develop a food allergy, connect with health experts who can educate and support you.

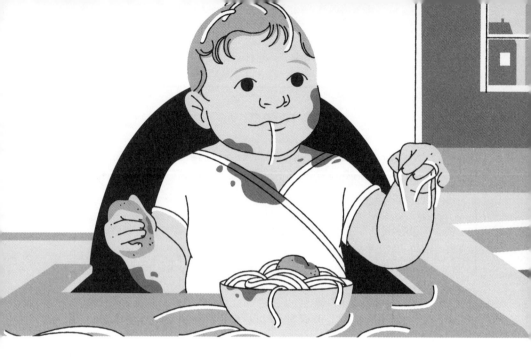

Chapter Fifteen

Nutrition for New Eaters

Every day, Maryam's mom was worried that she wasn't offering enough variety of food and that her baby wasn't eating enough of the solid foods she did offer. She was concerned her baby's nutrition, health, and development were all going to be negatively impacted, and even though Maryam's doctor said she was thriving, her mom shared that she still felt the need to urge baby Maryam to eat every last bite. She didn't trust herself or Maryam's feeding cues.

B abies are born with an internal system that helps them seek out food when they are hungry and stop when they are full. Baby's stomach communicates with their brain that it is empty, causing baby to feel hungry and seek food, or that it's full, causing baby to feel satisfied and stop eating.[1] This remarkable system is also influenced by a number of other internal and external factors, yet it typically works seamlessly for most infants.

There is typically no need to fret over how much food a baby is eating or not eating as they begin exploring solid foods. When you focus on the learnings of previous chapters (serving a variety of foods, letting baby explore without much pressure to consume, and sharing meals so you can model how to eat), nearly all babies learn to eat what they need and stop eating when they are full, which allows them to thrive. Let's dive in.

Hunger and Fullness Cues Start at the Breast or Bottle

Baby first learns to tap into their intuitive feelings of hunger and fullness and communicate what they feel with their breast or bottle feeds. Over time, baby hones their ability to recognize and respond to these cues, and as caregivers we learn to respond more appropriately. Everything comes together and despite the bumps and mistakes, baby eats what they need to grow and thrive, and we learn how to support baby in this. While this imperfect internal system can be temporarily overridden by other internal or external factors, like the need to poop or a very loud, cold, distracting room, most babies figure it out. We discuss this more later.

Signs of Hunger and Fullness

When baby is mainly relying on breast milk and formula for their nourishment, signs of hunger may look like the following:

→ turning their head toward the breast or bottle
→ sucking on their fists

→ puckering, smacking, or licking their lips

→ clenched hands and/or tensed body language

While many people associate a crying baby with hunger, not every cry is a sign of hunger. If a baby is crying because of hunger, it is likely long after baby signaled that they were ready to eat, and baby may now be overly hungry.[2,3] Signs of fullness may look like the following:

→ slowing down the pace of drinking

→ relaxing body and/or falling asleep during a feed

→ long pauses between sucking bursts

→ pushing the breast or bottle away

→ turning or shaking their head

→ distracted and more interested in surroundings

Research suggests that baby's cues of hunger and fullness may be more subtle than we expect, so keep an eye open for these signals and follow baby's lead.[4,5]

Hunger and Fullness with Solids

Baby has been developing the ability to listen to their feelings of hunger and fullness for months while bottle- and breastfeeding, and eventually they will apply those same skills to eating solids. But, it will take some time. When a baby comes to the table, they have a lot to learn—new skills to practice and many frustrating mistakes to work through. Showing up to the table when they are too hungry can lead to frustration. Their skills do not yet line up with their hunger needs, so baby will continue to rely on breast and bottle feeds to satisfy their hunger as they build their feeding skills.

At the table, look for signs of interest that let you know baby is ready to explore, and different signals that show they are at their limit.

As the weeks go by, baby will come to the table with you two and then three times per day and get more practice chewing, and eventually swallow more food. It will begin to click that food can *also* fill their belly and satisfy their hunger.

This positive feedback loop gradually strengthens over time to fuel baby's understanding that food provides pleasure, fullness, and satisfaction, eventually leading to baby eating more at the table. This tends to happen around 9 months of age, sometimes sooner and sometimes later. There is no need to rush baby to the finish line. Some babies may need a little extra support to explore solids with some gentle hunger by spacing out solids from the last breast or bottle feed, while others need more consistent practice while not hungry.

In toddlerhood, the child will transition to a mealtime schedule, moving away from "on demand" feeding, as they become more efficient at eating more at once and can go longer stretches between meals.

Honoring Baby's Intuition

Babies are born with all the tools their bodies need to develop the ability to listen and respond to feelings of hunger and fullness. The hormone ghrelin initiates feelings of hunger and a desire to eat. Once food has been consumed, the body recognizes the variety of foods eaten, feels the pressure of food in the stomach, and launches further hormonal signals to the gut and brain to communicate satisfaction and fullness. At that moment, baby will feel full, until the body gradually becomes hungry again, and the cycle repeats itself.[6,7,8,9,10]

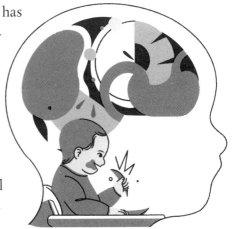

That said, signals of hunger and fullness can get crossed when a baby is sick and teething or when a toddler just can't get enough playtime. As parents and caregivers, our job is to gently remind, guide, and support our child in checking in with their body and internal cues to help them better listen to their needs for nourishment. Many children and adults need these gentle reminders, too—this is a journey of ongoing learning.

Feelings of fullness and satisfaction can also depend on what foods have been consumed. Having balanced meals with protein, fat, and carbohydrates can help promote a happy mood by triggering the brain to release serotonin and dopamine in response to the foods we eat.[11] In other words, balanced meals make our brains and bodies happy. Breast milk and formula *are* balanced meals for babies, so this applies for babies, toddlers, and beyond.

Despite this, the thought of letting a baby "just eat until they're full" can feel intimidating and scary. Research confirms that this is a common concern.[12] Many parents believe it's best for the parent to decide how much a baby or child should eat, and that making sure a baby is getting enough involves calculating nutrients and counting bites.

But it's not meant to be that way.

You can trust baby's ability to know when they are hungry or when they are full. If baby is signaling that they are hungry, let them eat, even if you think it's "too much." If baby is fussing and turning their head away, end the meal, even if you think they ate "too little." You can offer a breast or bottle feed after the meal if baby still seems hungry, but if baby refuses, that is okay, too.

What is normal for any baby or child to eat is extremely wide. If you follow any strict serving sizes or portions, you are likely to either underfeed or overfeed your child. Instead, take a responsive feeding approach, where we pay attention to baby's communication—interest, curiosity, hunger, and fullness cues—and offer opportunities to explore foods.[13] Research shows that taking a responsive feeding or intuitive eating approach helps support the whole family's relationship with food and their bodies.[14,15,16,17]

The only person who knows what's "enough" for baby's body is baby. And as long as they are tracking along their unique growth curve, happy, and otherwise thriving, then baby is likely receiving the nourishment they need.

Some children need more support because of medical conditions, sensory needs, and other factors, and benefit from working with a pediatric dietitian. Other children, like active and excited toddlers, may need reminders to check in with their bellies or some support through the discomfort of hunger or being overly full. Supporting your child in tuning in with their body will look different across life stages.

Factors Beyond Your Control That Influence Appetite

Many factors influence baby's appetite so it's completely normal for a baby's interest in food and the amount they eat to vary. Illness, teething, poor sleep, distractions, anxiousness, change of environment, being overly tired, and mealtime pressure and stress can decrease baby's appetite. Growth spurts, a delicious food, catching up after illness, and a more active day can increase appetite. Other factors such as certain medical conditions, force-feeding, food insecurity, stress, and trauma can disrupt this process of hunger and fullness communication.[18,19,20,21]

Understanding the "why" behind a shift in appetite can help if you're feeling worried. Issues such as illness and teething are temporary, and remembering this can help you feel less anxious when baby does not eat as much at mealtime.

Most blips in baby's appetite even out on their own. However, if baby's change in appetite persists for a few days to a week, or if you observe any of the following warning signs or have concerns, connect with baby's pediatric healthcare provider for guidance and reassurance.

Warning signs may include the following:

→ refusal of formula or breast milk for several feeds in a row
→ persistent refusal of solid food when the child was accepting it previously
→ reduced wet diapers (fewer than four full wet diapers in 24 hours, although this varies)
→ low energy or lethargy
→ inconsolable irritability
→ weight loss or difficulty gaining weight

Honoring Baby's Cues Amid Weight and Growth Concerns

Overly controlling how much a child eats can create challenges in feeding, as well as a child's ability to be guided by their feelings of hunger and fullness. Studies show that when parents try to pressure their children to eat more or less, it can lead to eating and appetite struggles, further refusals, aversion, mealtime battles, food fixations, and even social-emotional consequences, like food shame or guilt.[22,23,24,25,26,27]

The drive to control how much food a child eats can often be traced back to beliefs many of us have been taught around body image, weight, and health. Sometimes your success as a parent or caregiver feels related to a child's weight on the scale.

For example, the belief that a child's body doesn't look as it "should" can increase stress, leading to changed behaviors around feeding—such as pushing baby to eat more or restricting them to eat less. This can build a challenging foundation for baby's body image in the longer term. This negative internal dialogue may look like, "Baby isn't eating enough, that's why they're not gaining enough, and that's why they're not as filled out as other babies. I need to get my baby to eat more." This can hurt mealtime dynamics and lead to decreased interest in eating over time as the child's own communication of their body's needs are overridden and ignored.[28] It can also carry on for years, and the older child may be less motivated to come to the dinner table and may feel that they are too small, or too big, or undesirable by other people's standards, or that their hunger cues are not to be trusted.[29]

In supporting baby, it is helpful to think about our own beliefs around food and body image. If you have concerns about baby's size and are tempted to shift how you feed your baby as a result, take a step back and a deep breath. Remember that baby is more than capable of communicating what they need, and you are more than capable of listening.

Nutrition by Age

When babies start showing signs of readiness for solid foods, usually around 6 months of age, you can start by offering baby one meal at the table. Aim to offer a variety of food groups and textures, including iron-rich foods such as meat, poultry, seafood, beans, nuts, and seeds, prepared in developmentally appropriate ways. At this time many babies may not be eating a significant amount of solid food. That is entirely fine; breast milk and formula will be providing the bulk of baby's nutrition as they explore the road to solid foods.

Around 8 to 9 months of age, you can increase to two meals per day. Continue to offer a variety of food groups and textures. When it comes to navigating the transition from breast milk and formula to solid foods, there's no need to deliberately reduce breast milk or formula. Baby's nursing sessions and bottles continue to be similar as they were before, as baby decides how much solids to eat.

Around 10 to 11 months of age, as baby's feeding skills progress, baby can be offered meals two to three times per day.[30] The amount of breast milk and formula a baby eats may decrease slightly at this time, or baby may continue to consume similar amounts as before; both are completely fine. In either case, breast milk and formula will continue to act as their nutritional safety net.

At 12 months, baby is now a toddler who has gotten better at feeding themselves, and we expect that they will gradually drink less breast milk and formula around 12 to 15 months of age, as they increasingly consume solid foods. This will look different for every child and the exact timing varies. Keep in mind that cow's milk is not meant to replace formula or breast milk. At this age, your toddler will likely be joining and eating the family meals and continuing to experience a variety of nourishing foods.

By 12 to 15 months of age, most children receive the majority of their nutrition from solid foods. There is no need to rush to the finish line. Trust the process, continue to create a positive eating environment, offer a variety of foods, and expect a nonlinear journey. Some babies and toddlers need more time to figure things out; others less. With time, you'll have a self-feeding toddler.

For families offering primarily formula feeds and whose babies have progressed to a varied diet by 12 to 15 months of age, feel free to wean off formula. The child can transition to cow's milk or another calcium-fortified milk alternative as a beverage, if needed, or a child may choose not to drink milk at all. As long as a child has a varied diet with plenty of sources of protein, fat, and calcium, such as yogurt, cheese, and tofu, cow's milk isn't actually a requirement for many toddlers.

Many families continue breastfeeding their toddlers for months to years after infancy. Keep in mind that solids are the main source of nutrition for toddlers, so aim to space out nursing sessions so that the toddler is hungry at mealtimes. Families who are ready to stop breastfeeding can also transition to cow's milk or another calcium-fortified milk alternative, or they can skip the cow's milk entirely.

Building a Balanced Plate for Baby

A plate of nourishing food for baby looks a lot like a balanced plate for an adult, just smaller, with food that is cooked and cut for baby's age and developmental ability. Just like adults, babies need meals that contain a variety of food groups that provide carbohydrates, proteins, fats, and other important nutrients. Since babies are growing and developing so rapidly at this stage, they have higher fat needs than adults.[31]

When it comes to making meals for baby, offer a range and selection of a variety of foods throughout the week. Aim to provide foods such as grains, proteins, fats, and fruits and vegetables—but keep it simple. Invite yourself to embrace the art of "good enough" when it comes to preparing meals for baby.

Breaking Down Nutrition

We have all heard of different nutrients, vitamins, and minerals. But what are they and what do they do in our bodies? Read on as we break down important nutrients for you and baby.

Carbohydrates: Carbohydrates (such as grains, potatoes, and fruits) provide a source of energy to fuel baby's developing brain, crawling, and endless curiosity. Fiber is also a type of carbohydrate that supports digestion, the growth of healthy intestinal bacteria, and regular bowel movements.

Fat: More than 50 percent of a baby's nutritional needs come from fat, whether it's from breast milk, formula, solid foods, or a combination of all three.[32] Fat provides a dense form of energy and a sense of lasting fullness and satisfaction between feeds and meals. Fat can be found in oils, butter, cheese, nuts, seeds, seafood, meat, and poultry (as well as in breast milk and formula). Omega-3 fatty acids (commonly found in seafood, nuts, and seeds) are a form of fat that helps support brain development, vision, immune function, and other bodily functions.

Protein: Protein also plays a role in helping the body feel full and satisfied while providing lasting energy. It fuels developing muscles, supports the immune system, and more. While many parents worry that their baby isn't receiving "enough protein," protein is present in a wide variety of foods, such as formula, breast milk, dairy products, meat, poultry, eggs, seafood, beans, nuts, seeds, and certain grains and vegetables.

Iron: Around 6 months of age, baby's iron stores naturally become decreased, and baby needs iron from solid foods. Focus on regularly offering iron-rich foods, and trust that, with practice and time, baby will get the iron they need from the food they eat. Iron comes in heme (animal-based) and nonheme (plant-based) forms. Heme iron is more readily absorbed than nonheme; however, pairing nonheme iron foods with those rich in vitamin C, like fruits and vegetables, can help boost iron absorption.

Iron supports healthy red blood cells, neurodevelopment, focus, mood, sleep quality, and more. Iron deficiency is the most common nutrient deficiency in the world and significantly impacts children under 5 years of age.[33] Many factors influence a child's iron status, such as being born preterm or term, medications, and certain medical conditions. Some babies need iron supplements, despite consuming iron-rich foods, and that is exactly what they are there for. A common worry with self-feeding is that baby will not consume enough iron; however, a study from 2017 found that as long as babies were offered iron-rich foods with most meals, there was minimal difference in iron status between self-feeding babies and traditionally spoon-fed babies.[34] For a list of iron-rich foods, see Chapter 9.

Zinc: Similarly to iron, baby's zinc stores also become decreased around 6 months of age, meaning that baby also needs zinc from solid foods. Zinc supports immune function, taste and smell perception, wound healing, growth and development, and more. Most iron-rich foods are also rich in zinc, such as meat, poultry, seafood, and eggs, as well as beans, nuts, and seeds.

Vitamins A, B, C, and D: Vitamin A and its many different forms support vision, skin health, and immunity. It can be found in most fruits, vegetables, fatty fish, and dairy products. Eight different B vitamins play important roles in supporting metabolic processes, energy, red blood cell health, and more. B vitamins can be found in a wide variety of foods including legumes, grains, proteins, and fruits and vegetables. Vitamin C is found in most fruits and vegetables. In addition to supporting immunity and skin health, it also helps boost non-heme (plant-based) iron absorption. Lastly, vitamin D supports bone health, hormone health, and more, but it is not found in many foods, and it is commonly supplemented in babies to support adequate levels in the body. The foods it is encountered in include fatty fish, UV-exposed mushrooms, eggs, and certain dairy products.

This is just a snapshot of a few vital nutrients for baby's growth and development. Unless baby's diet is restricted, most babies can obtain these nutrients and others by offering a variety of foods and doing your best.

Cow's Milk, Dairy, and Calcium Considerations

Around 12 months of age, cow's milk may be offered to most toddlers. Just keep in mind that cow's milk is not meant as an ounce-for-ounce replacement for breast milk or formula. The majority of the toddler's nourishment will be coming from solid foods, and milk is a beverage to accompany a meal. Aim for 16 oz (480 mL) or less per day. It is not necessary to offer cow's milk—the nutrients in cow's milk are found in many foods, like cheese, yogurt, fish, and calcium-fortified milk-alternative products, as well as in plant-based sources (such as sesame, almonds, and certain dark leafy greens). Some kids can fill up on too much milk, decreasing their drive for solids and increasing the risk of iron deficiency, poor appetite, constipation, and challenges with growth.[35,36] Setting gentle boundaries helps provide the guidance that children need to avoid filling up on any one kind of food in excess, so they can achieve the balance they need to thrive.

Signs of Nourishment

The amount of food baby eats can vary widely from day to day. We suggest paying more attention to what baby eats over a whole week instead of a single day. Often, a refused dinner leads to a larger interest in breakfast the following morning. Most babies have an excellent sense of just how much milk and solid food they need to not only thrive but grow into the body size that their genetic potential is guiding and that their body is happiest at.

A common concern for many is how to determine if baby is receiving "enough" nutrition. Fortunately, there are a few simple ways to know if your baby is getting what they need to grow, develop, and thrive. Many of these points are easily observable at home—no fancy tests or equipment necessary.

✓ Baby is taking in relatively consistent amounts of breast milk or formula (expect natural variations due to colds, teething, and other situations). If baby is eating enough, you can expect them to be making numerous wet diapers daily and pooping comfortably.

✓ Baby is happily, curiously, and energetically exploring their world and environment.

✓ Baby is learning new skills and developing as expected.

✓ Baby is growing and gaining weight appropriately.

✓ Baby is sleeping well (within reason for their age and development).

How Much Food Is Enough? How Much Is Too Much?

One of the most common questions parents and caregivers ask is "How much food should I offer baby?" and "How do I know baby consumed enough?"

Surprisingly enough, most babies will be looking internally for that answer, so you can watch them, trust them, and learn their cues for hunger and fullness to see how much is "just right." Learning to respond to hunger and fullness cues takes time and practice, and mistakes are all a part of the process.

As we've discussed throughout the book, it takes time for babies to learn the complex and important act of self-feeding and how to respond to their hunger and fullness cues appropriately. Most importantly, every baby is different, and this journey can vary from child to child. Some babies are enthusiastic eaters. Others are slower to warm up to solid foods. Both are completely fine and totally normal.

For many parents and caregivers, it can be helpful to visualize how much food to start baby's meal with; look to offer about a quarter of a typical adult portion of food. Keep any extra food in sight so baby can reach or grunt for it. If baby wants more, offer more. If they're no longer showing interest in the food, it's fine to end the meal and try again at the next one.

If baby is tired, sick, or teething, they may not want to eat solids at all, and that's okay. If they want to stop, stop.

If baby is going through a growth spurt or had a lot of physical activity that day, they may want to eat a lot. If baby wants more, offer more. Simple as that. Many parents are fearful that "too much" food could lead to digestive issues or growth concerns, but most babies know just when to stop for their individual needs.

In fact, it's generally unusual for babies to eat "too much," and even if they truly did, every instance of "overeating" is actually a learning opportunity to explore and understand the shifting boundaries of the body. While overeating may not feel great in the moment, it is temporary and passing and comes with a learning occasion. Let baby experiment and figure out concepts of cause and effect with the ways that food can make their body feel.

In some cases, babies with certain medical conditions, feeding difficulties, and other circumstances may need more help and assistance in receiving the nourishment they need to thrive. Working with pediatric nutrition and feeding specialists can help these children find ways to nourish their bodies in ways that feel best for them.

> Maryam's mom was surprised to learn that she was actually doing an amazing job—she just didn't realize it. She didn't know that she could offer her daughter and herself grace and flexibility in the journey to eating solids. From then on, she felt a lot more relaxed at the table, knowing that simply offering variety, moving flexibly with the demands of life, and honoring her baby's readiness and interest in solid foods are the best things that she could do—and that was more than enough.

Joy Is Nourishment

The feelings we have around food, our connection to family and cultural traditions, and the pleasure we take in each other's company are just as important as the foods we eat and the nutrition our bodies receive. Remember, joy is part of a nourishing diet, too.

Heavy Metals in Food

Every other day, it feels like there is a headline in the news about heavy metals in our foods. Parents can't help but worry if the foods they're offering their babies are safe—and where do these heavy metals even come from?

Heavy metals, such as arsenic, cadmium, lead, and mercury, make their way into soil and water through the use of certain pesticides, mining activities, pollution, and other human activities. As a result, heavy metals are absorbed by foods grown in soil and by seafood and sea plants in the ocean. The amount of heavy metals absorbed in a food will vary by location, the food at hand, and the degree of heavy metal contamination in a given area; this applies to both organic and conventionally produced foods.

The reality (and we know this is unsettling) is that the majority of the foods we eat have some degree of heavy metal contamination. And while regularly consuming too much of a food that contains excess heavy metals may impact a child's health, growth, and development, it's important to take a balanced approach. Most parents are reassured to know that exposure to heavy metals is limited when we allow baby to practice feeding themselves, and we offer a variety of foods over mealtimes. To further reduce exposure to heavy metals, try to reduce or avoid fish high in mercury, serve fruit instead of fruit juice, offer a variety of grains in addition to or instead of infant rice cereal, and make sure water sources used for cooking and drinking are regularly tested and deemed safe for use. Additionally, you can aim to serve baby a variety of nutrient-rich foods, especially foods that are rich in calcium, iron, protein, vitamin C, and zinc, which help reduce the absorption and negative impacts of heavy metals.[37,38,39,40,41]

Can Babies Have Salt and Sugar?

One of the most confusing and polarizing aspects of navigating nutrition for baby is added sugar and salt in baby's food.

We summarize the research simply as this: Baby can eat food containing salt and added sugar as part of a variety of foods in the diet. There is no strong research to support the idea that baby having an occasional taste of food with salt and/or sugar is dangerous.[42,43] The goal is to aim for a realistic balance: Reduce added sugar and salt when it makes sense, and when it is not possible, enjoy your meal and move on with your day, keeping the long game in mind. If you are worried, remember: Most babies naturally limit the amount of food consumed at any given meal because they are still figuring out how food works, and this naturally limits how much salt or sugar is eaten at first.

If you are wondering what the research says:

- A recent literature review suggests that there is not enough evidence to make the claim that sodium intake in infancy alone is associated with blood pressure, cardiac, or kidney problems later in life.[44,45,46]
- In fact, restricting sodium and sugar was associated with younger children seeking out salty and sugary foods, compared to children who already had these foods in their diet.[47,48,49,50,51]
- If there is a risk, it may be related to long-term health: some studies suggest that regularly eating excessive amounts of food that is very high in sodium and sugar in early life (such as juice, soda, and salty and sweetened snacks) may impact health later in life, such as increasing the risk of cavities or decreasing the variety of foods consumed over time.[52,53]

When you want to serve baby's food without or with less added salt or sugar, there is no need to prepare a special meal for baby. Instead, it might look like this: prepare a meal as you normally would do for yourself, hold off on adding salt or sugar (or reduce it), set aside a portion for baby, and season the rest of the food as you would for yourself. Fortunately, a dash of added salt or sugar here and there is not going to make or break baby's health. For many families, taking a flexible approach provides more opportunities to share a wider variety of foods with their babies than they otherwise would have—and the peace of mind and confidence to do so. Remember that nutrition perfectionism is not our goal. No meal or food is truly ever "perfect."[54]

Vitamins and Supplements

Contrary to popular belief, not all babies need nutritional supplements; that's why an individualized approach is essential. In the United States, vitamin D is often prescribed for exclusively breastfed infants, a vitamin K injection is recommended at birth, and iron supplementation is sometimes prescribed. Generally, typically developing children who consume a varied diet don't need additional supplements, although those with restricted diets, allergies, or medical conditions may require them. Ultimately, consulting a pediatrician or pediatric dietitian can help provide personalized advice regarding supplements.

How Much Should Baby Weigh?

This is one of the most common questions parents have, and to the surprise of many, there is no one right answer. As parents, we cannot help but compare our baby to others. Is my baby growing too fast? Too slow? Is it normal for my 4-month-old baby to be in 9-month-old clothes? Is it normal for my 6-month-old baby to still be in 3-month-old clothes?

When we examine weight on a day-to-day basis, we find that over the first 3 to 4 months of life, most babies gain between 20 and 30 grams per day, on average. Weight gain then decreases to an average of 15 to 20 grams per day for the remainder of the first year of life. Some babies gain more, others less, but both are normal. Weight gain is anything but perfectly linear, and, like infant growth, it happens over a period of time. Day-to-day fluctuations are expected and normal.

You may be wondering, "How do we know when baby is gaining

adequate weight if we are not supposed to weigh them daily?" This is where growth charts can come in handy.

What Are Growth Charts?

A growth chart is a tool that is used to track a child's weight, length, and head circumference measurements over a period of time to help track overall growth patterns. Growth charts are broken down by biological sex, as differences in linear growth and weight gain are already present in early infancy. There are also growth charts for children with special medical needs such as prematurity or Down syndrome.

The key word here is "pattern." Growth charts are not designed to analyze normal day-to-day fluctuations; it is the child's pattern of growth over time that is of interest. Small changes from one day, one week, or even one month to the next are generally not a cause for concern. The percentile isn't a grade—your child doesn't need to jump to higher percentiles, and there is no perfect percentile to be at. If they're at the 1st percentile and growing along their curve, that's great. If they're at the 99th percentile and growing along their curve, that's great. There is a misunderstanding that being either high or at the middle is "ideal." Children's bodies come in a wide range of healthy, happy, and beautiful shapes and sizes.

Growth charts help illustrate a child's pattern of growth over time and give us a sense of what is normal for that child. But conclusions about a child's overall health status should never be made in isolation by using the data a growth chart provides.

Are Growth Charts Accurate?

Obtaining accurate and precise measurements in young children is difficult and often done incorrectly. When it comes to infants, variables such as a wet versus dry diaper, different office scales, clothed versus unclothed, wiggling on the scale, and a recent feed or an empty

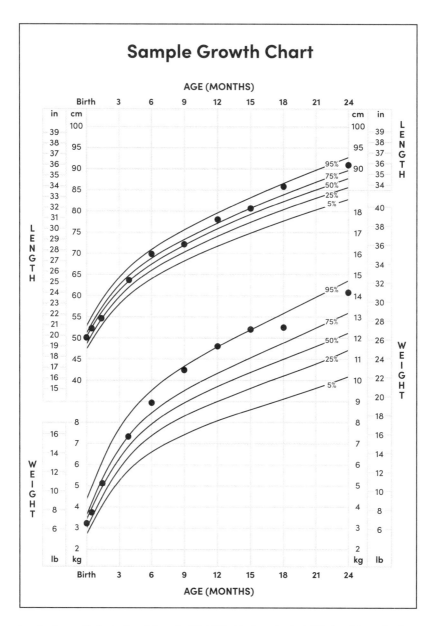

A patient's growth chart adapted from the World Health Organization's "Birth to 24 months: Boys length-for-age percentiles and weight-for-age percentiles" growth chart. Note how the child crosses several different percentiles during the first 24 months of life.

tummy can all skew a baby's weight higher or lower, depending on the timing and the situation. The same applies to length, where a squirmy baby can affect the accuracy of length measurements, which in turn can greatly skew weight-for-length measurements. It's important to understand the factors that go into weight and length measurements so you can understand what an accurate measurement is (and avoid unnecessary stress when the numbers may look off).

That said, fluctuations in weight and height, whether from growth spurts, illnesses, teething, and more, are also normal and to be expected. For this reason, it is important to examine growth charts in context.

Examining a Growth Chart Together

Let's look at a growth chart on page 231 for 0 to 24 months of age. The patient is a male child, born full term, with no known medical conditions. The dots may seem overwhelming at first, so let's get oriented. Along the horizontal axis is the child's age over time in 3 month intervals. Along the vertical axis we see weight (in pounds and kilograms) on the bottom half and length (in inches and centimeters) on the top half. The curved lines that run across the graph represent percentiles between the 5th and 95th percentiles.

Let's test ourselves: What were this child's weight and length percentiles at 15 months?

95th percentile for weight (about 12.5 kg or 27.5 lb)

75th percentile for length (about 81 cm or 31.9 inches)

When we look at this child's weight over time, you may notice that this child touched several different weight percentiles, ranging between the 40th and 95th percentiles. He is also at or above the 90th percentile with respect to weight. Is this good? Is this bad?

It's neither, it just is. He is following his own curve from a weight and length perspective beautifully. He doubled his birth weight before 4 months of age and tripled his birth weight before 9 months. Is this a cause for alarm? If you ask his mother, she will tell you that he started self-feeding around 6 months of age and has been a very enthusiastic eater. Between 15 and 18 months of age, he doesn't seem to gain any weight. Is this normal? It can be, but we need more information. His mother will tell you that he began walking around 13 months of age but really didn't start moving until 15 months of age, and since then he has been nonstop. So little to no weight gain is completely normal given the significantly increased physical activity. If the mother said that he has been experiencing very watery bowel movements for the past two weeks and has been feeling ill, low energy, or otherwise "off" from his baseline health, this would warrant further investigation. There is no specific percentile or number that baby should strive for. A child can be healthy at nearly any size. The main goal of any growth chart is to observe weight and length measurements that follow a relatively consistent pattern over time. And remember, when interpreting growth charts, it's *always* important to take a step back and look at the child's overall health.

Warning Signs

If your child experiences any of the following symptoms, or if you have any concerns, please reach out to their primary care provider immediately. Support from other specialists, such as pediatric dietitians, feeding therapists, endocrinologists, and gastroenterologists, may be warranted.

- Long-term decreases in weight and/or length percentiles. This may appear like a flat line on a growth chart with little to no increase in weight or length or a declining trend.

- Clothing fitting looser

- Unexplained and chronically decreased appetite

- Unexplained and chronically decreased energy

- Decreased interest and engagement in playing

- Refusal to eat or drink for several meals in a row

- Sleeping much more than usual

- Reduced number of wet diapers (especially if fewer than 4 full diapers per 24 hours)

Patterns Matter More Than Percentiles

Growth charts, while helpful over the long term, can be inaccurate and misinterpreted by clinicians and parents alike. They are simply a tool that's designed to be used to collect data and are not meant to be interpreted on their own without context.[55,56,57,58] You do not need to obsess over your child's weight or length percentiles. Use your loving attention instead to tune in to your child's hunger cues, honor their signals for when they are done, and provide an overall nurturing environment.

Summary

✓ Most babies are born with the tools they need to intuitively eat enough food to thrive; there's no need to pressure baby to take "one more bite" or to restrict food.

✓ When it comes to building a meal for baby, offer a variety of foods and embrace the art of "good enough" with mealtimes.

✓ Aim to offer iron-rich foods with most meals to help support baby's energy, development, and iron stores.

✓ When it comes to added salt and sugar, reduce where you can, don't stress where you can't, and know that if you offer a variety of foods and create joyful meals, baby will be just fine.

✓ Babies and children come in a wide range of healthy shapes and sizes.

✓ When interpreting growth charts, context matters. A recent illness, growth spurt, or transition to walking can all influence growth measurements.

✓ If growth patterns suggest that baby needs more support, trust that their healthcare team will inform you. If you're worried, express your concerns.

✓ Fluctuations in weight are normal. They can happen for many reasons, like illness and teething. Most babies get back on rhythm once they're feeling better.

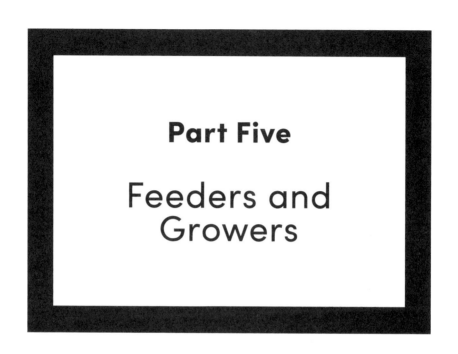

Part Five

Feeders and Growers

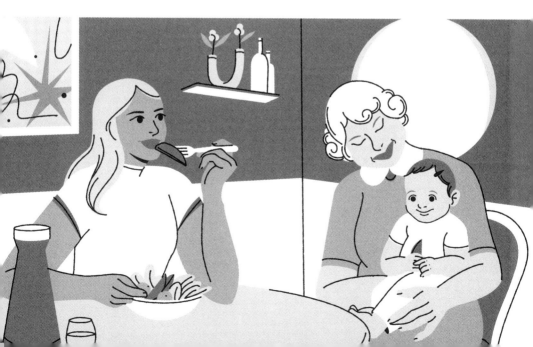

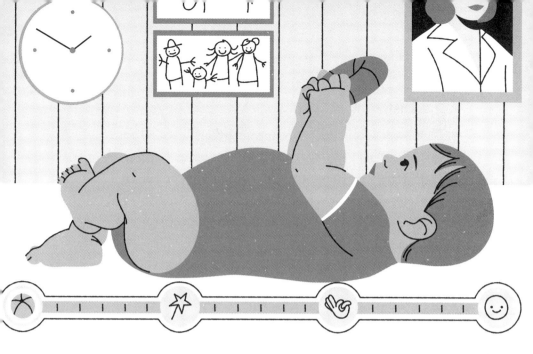

Chapter Sixteen

Prep Time
(4 to 5 Months)

I t's time to talk about what you can do to support baby's development (and feeding skills along the way!). If you are ever concerned
about baby's development, bring it up to their healthcare provider.
Accessible developmental support through early intervention programs is available for most families.

Use the following checklist to keep track of the things you can be
doing with baby to support their development during this valuable
prep time.

Checklist

- ☐ Provide lots of floor time to strengthen neck and core.
- ☐ Include baby in your mealtimes as often as possible.
- ☐ Prepare your home and get your gear (high chair, etc.).
- ☐ Determine whether baby is at high risk of food allergies.
- ☐ Take an infant CPR and choking first aid class.
- ☐ Review signs of readiness for solid food.
- ☐ Get on the same page with your caregivers. Discuss goals and pace for how you'd like to start solids.

We call the 4- to 5-month age range "prep time" because it's exactly that: time for baby to develop some foundational skills that will prepare them to practice eating solid food once they are ready to start. There is not a lot you need to do beyond putting baby in the right environment to play and move, and observing baby to notice the small but significant new skills that naturally emerge when babies are allowed to play and explore.

Developmental Milestones

This is a favorite time for many parents, as their newborns start to come out of their shell, express themselves more, stay awake longer, and begin to interact with their environment. It's also a period known for broken sleep and tired parents as a baby's sleep cycles begin to change and mature. Following are some of the developmental milestones you can expect to see from baby during this time.[1,2,3]

Gross Motor Skills

- → Starting to hold head up
- → Looking from side to side
- → Pushing body up/moving arms against gravity
- → Beginning to sit up

At this age, most babies really start moving their body and holding up their head with more control. While on their back, they look from side to side and start kicking their legs and moving their arms against gravity. While on their belly, many babies can lift their head up off the ground and look around. They may start to prop themselves up on their elbows while looking around, and as baby gets closer to 6 months of age, they will begin to push up higher on fully extended arms. Around 4 months of age, while baby is sitting on your lap, their spine will still be a bit rounded, but they will start to extend and sit up straighter as their core muscles continue to get stronger. You will likely see baby starting to figure out how to roll.

Fine Motor Skills

→ Hands staying open more, fingers and thumb stretching out
→ Grabbing large objects
→ Waving or shaking toys
→ Bringing objects to their mouth

Babies in this time frame are starting to learn that their hands can do a lot of fun things. While many babies still remain fisted around 4 months, you'll likely see their hands staying open more often, stretching out those fingers and thumb. By 5 months of age, baby should be able to more flexibly open their fingers and bat at and try to grab larger objects with their hands. They can bring their hands together in the middle while on their back and on their side and will play with their fingers. They can hold a toy that is placed in their hand, and some may even wave or shake the toy a bit. They will also start bringing their hands, and toys placed in their hands, to their mouth. While on their back or on their side, they start to actively reach for items that are held in front of them or overhead.

Cognitive/Language/Social-Emotional Skills

→ Smiling

→ Making sounds, sometimes laughing or babbling

→ Tracking objects (or you) when moving side to side

→ Turning head toward sound

Infants begin interacting more with the world during this time. You'll notice that baby makes better eye contact with you and will even track toys or your face when moving from side to side. They enjoy visually inspecting things that are placed in their hands or in their field of vision. They will turn their head toward sounds and respond positively when they hear the voice of a familiar caregiver. Many parents feel that their baby is easier to calm at this age, and some get very good at using a pacifier or their hands for support when they are upset.

Activities for 4- to 5-Month-Olds

Young babies find almost anything interesting, so you do not need any special toys or tools to help grow baby's skills during prep time. We will share motor activities that strengthen the muscles that are important for coming to the table in the next few months and other activities that specifically strengthen baby's ability to imitate, pay attention, and problem solve—all of which will come in handy at the table and beyond. We'll focus specifically on some key prefeeding activities that can set baby up for success with the next step of starting solid foods.

Motor Activities

Often called "unrestricted floor time," placing baby on their back on a soft blanket on a flat surface allows them to move, reach, stretch, push off, roll, look around, and explore their environment. Floor time builds strength in the neck, arms, belly, and back and helps develop body awareness—knowing where the body is in space—which is the building block of coordinated motor movements.

Car seats, bouncy chairs, Bumbo seats, and other infant containers keep baby relatively still, limiting exploration and movement options. The more time a baby spends on the floor in comparison to in sitting devices, the more their muscles have a chance to practice moving and build skill.

Floor time play does not have to be complicated. Find a safe area of your home, place a soft blanket on the floor, and give baby opportunities to lie in all three positions: on their back, on their side, and on their belly. Once they can roll, there's no need to move them into the different positions; let them choose where they would like to play.

→ With baby lying on their back, roll a small towel or blanket and place it under baby's hips to elevate them slightly. This can help baby reach for their feet and use their tummy muscles.

→ Place ring toys or noise-making socks on baby's feet to encourage reaching for the feet.

→ If baby is reaching for an item, place it slightly out of reach to encourage rolling to the side to retrieve it.

→ Some babies love tummy time; you can either place them on the floor on their belly easily or start on their back and gently roll them over.

→ When on their belly, give baby something to look at. Set up toys, books, or black-and-white cards in front of them, or even get down on the floor and smile and talk to baby.

→ Lay baby on their side and use a towel roll behind their back to help them stay there, then place a toy just out of baby's reach, so they use their arms to try to get it. You can even gently tap baby's arm with the toy to encourage them to reach for it.

Cognitive Activities

Here are a few ways to specifically work on baby's attention, imitation, problem-solving skills, and language skills. The more language exposure baby has in that first year the better, and you can do a few specific things to draw baby in and improve their attention, imitation, turn-taking skills, and connection with you.[4,5,6]

→ **Face-to-face mirroring:** Sit with baby on your lap, with their back on your legs, so they are looking up at your face. Wait for baby to look up at you, then use facial expressions to mimic what you see baby do. After a few minutes, try to get baby to imitate you. You can smile, open your mouth, blink your eyes, stick out your tongue, or blow raspberries.

→ **Talk and sing:** Get baby face-to-face and have a conversation or sing some simple songs to them. Try starting then pausing for a few seconds to see if baby waits for you to keep going.

→ **Turn-taking:** Anytime baby makes a sound or does a specific motion, such as tapping on a tray, imitate the noise or action they make. Go back and forth if baby is interested.

→ **Problem-solving games:** Partially cover a toy with a small blanket and ask, "Where's the toy?" After a few seconds, uncover the toy, explaining, "There it is!" Re-cover it partially and wait for baby to try to find it on their own.

Prefeeding Activities and Sensory Activities

There are a few activities that you can add into your day that help expose baby to food, mealtimes, and eating before they even take their first bite.

→ Bring baby to the table or around food even though they aren't eating. Let baby watch you eat, cook, and taste food in the kitchen. If you'd like, you can narrate what is happening: "I'm tasting Grandma's delicious tomato soup!" Babies show interest in the things that adults enjoy (cellphones, keys!), so demonstrate to baby that mealtimes are fun by smiling, laughing, and engaging with food and your family around the dinner table. Make meals a place baby *wants* to be.

→ Allow baby to put their hands and toys in their mouth: babies poking the inside of their mouths with their hands and toys makes the gag reflex less sensitive and prepping the brain for something new to be in there very soon (solids). You may have heard of oral stimulation toys for babies. While these therapy tools are not necessary, they can be fun teethers if you'd like to offer them.

→ Avoid baby mittens: baby needs to explore their environment with their hands.

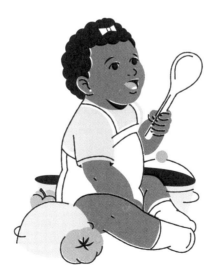

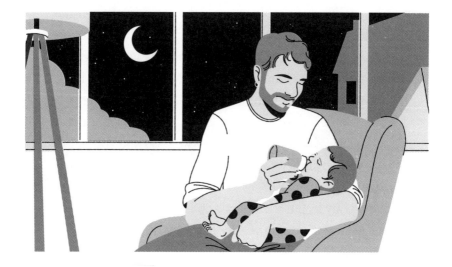

Schedules During Prep Time

Around this age, baby's day may be getting into a more predictable rhythm, but for some, each day may still be in flux. Most babies have figured out the difference between night and day by this time and continue to wake and feed during the night. Many babies in this age group are awake for about 1½ to 2 hours at a time, and take three or four naps per day.

Some like to follow a more specific schedule, while others follow more of a daily rhythm. Try to structure the day to give baby opportunities for rest, playtime, and feeding. There is no need to implement a firm schedule, and some babies do best with less rigidity in their daily routines; however, a flexible but consistent daily routine is helpful for both baby and parents.

Oral Hygiene

You don't have to wait for the first tooth to pop to start practicing oral hygiene. It can help early on to introduce a soft-bristled toothbrush to gently brush baby's gums to get them used to the sensation. Oral hygiene can even be performed with a soft cloth, gently rubbing along the gums. Focus on keeping this experience positive and aim for once a day.

Food and Nutrition During Prep Time

Unless you have been advised by your doctor to start solids early for exposure to a food allergen (e.g., for an infant at high risk of peanut or egg allergy) or there is some extenuating medical condition, the only food your baby needs at this age is breast milk or formula.

Many 4- to 5-month-old babies nurse 8 to 12 times per day, with some nursing a bit less, and most still nursing during the night. If taking bottles, baby will typically take 24 to 32 ounces (720 to 960 mL)—sometimes more, sometimes less—of breast milk or formula (or a mix) across 6 to 8 feeds (or more), and likely still takes bottles during the night. Many babies may also be taking vitamin D drops as recommended by their care provider. For more on vitamin D and supplements, see Chapter 15.

If you are breastfeeding or expressing breast milk, it's important to pump anytime baby is taking a bottle and when you are away from baby, in order to maintain your milk supply. Some babies become very distracted while nursing or bottle-feeding at this age, pulling off the breast or bottle and looking at anything somewhat interesting in their environment. If directly nursing, this can impact breast milk supply if it's happening consistently. If you notice that baby is very distracted, you may want to try to feed in a darker, very quiet room, and some people wear a necklace for baby to reach for and play with to keep them more focused. You may also need to feed baby more frequently to make up for this distraction.

Summary

✓ Babies 4 to 5 months old are becoming more aware of their surroundings, which makes this an excellent time to help prepare baby for starting solids.

✓ Focus on play activities that build baby's core strength and hand-eye coordination to set them up for success at the table in the months to come.

✓ While it may be too early to start solids, bringing your 4- to 5-month-old to the table or into the kitchen while you eat is a great way to increase their awareness and tolerance of the sights and smells of the family meal.

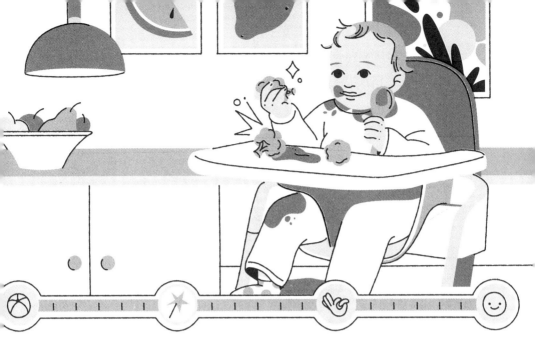

Chapter Seventeen

The Magic Window
(6 to 8 Months)

You've made it to the magic window! This is where all the fun starts. During this time, babies can begin to share the foods you are eating. They start learning to bring food to their mouth, practice chewing and moving food around to swallow—and you are learning how to eat with baby. At this age, babies are also blossoming into their own person, with new skills, tons of movement, and funny faces.[1]

During the transition to solid food, it's common for babies to figure out a certain movement or skill, and then stop doing it for a period of time, but come back to it at the next meal. This is normal. But remember, babies develop on their own timeline, and there is a range of normal for when these skills emerge. If you ever feel concerned about your child's development, bring it up with their healthcare provider.

Use the following checklist to keep track of the things you can be doing with baby to support their development during this window.[2,3,4]

Checklist

☐ Set up your high chair or seating system and adjust it as needed (more in Chapter 8).

☐ Review infant choking rescue and CPR.

☐ Think about your daily schedule, when solids will fit into your day, and what family foods you'd like to offer.

☐ Introduce common allergens such as peanut and egg.

☐ Introduce a variety of food flavors, textures, and colors, including foods that are rich in iron.

☐ Offer finger foods and let baby practice feeding themselves by 8 months of age.

☐ Make mealtime a joyful, fun place to be!

Developmental Milestones

During the Magic Window, babies start to really move. It's a common time for parenting to get more challenging as baby begins to move more freely around the environment and requires much more direct supervision. A common time for babyproofing the home, the Magic Window has its share of new challenges and fun milestones, one of which is starting solids.

Here are some of the developmental milestones you can expect to see from most babies during this time.

Gross Motor Skills

→ Crawling (some)
→ Rolling

→ Sitting
→ Scooting

By 6 months of age, most babies have figured out how to roll. Many have discovered that they can keep rolling over and over to get from one side of a room to the other. Baby may be scooting and rotating their body while on their back or tummy, and they can push their chest and shoulders up quite high using their hands and arms while in tummy time. By 7 or 8 months of age, many babies are starting to figure out how to crawl. While most 6-month-olds can keep their head, neck, and trunk upright when seated with a little support, many won't figure out how to get their body into and out of a seated position until closer to 7, 8, or even 9 months of age.

Fine Motor Skills

→ Discovering the hands
→ Reaching for and grabbing objects
→ Passing items back and forth

During this period, most babies discover their hands and all that they can do. Many have figured out that they can reach for items and grab them with one or both hands. Many babies can hold their own bottle, put a pacifier back in their mouth, and pass items back and forth between their hands. While many 6-month-olds can successfully grab and hold on to an item, gracefully releasing an item will come closer to 7 or 8 months of age. Most 6- to 8-month-olds will use their whole hand to grab large items.

Cognitive/Language/Social-Emotional Skills

→ Reaching for toys with intent
→ Developing basic problem-solving skills
→ Babbling in response to you

During this time, babies are discovering that they are a part of the world and that they can reach out, explore, and impact their environment. They reach for toys, try to move their body to get at things, and pick things up and bring them to their mouth to explore and learn. Babies this age are just starting to use basic problem-solving skills to figure out how things work and to get what they want. During this phase, many babies begin to babble back and forth with you.

Activities for 6- to 8-Month-Olds

Babies continue to be interested in almost anything during the Magic Window, and the activities outlined in the previous chapter continue to be great for a baby in the Magic Window, too. Here are more ideas to build baby's self-feeding skills.

Play Activities

→ Place toys on low surfaces in your home to give baby a reason to want to reach out or practice transitioning into sitting.

→ Let baby pick up medium-size items and drop them into a bucket or box.

→ Offer cubes, blocks, large puzzles, push-button toys, ring stackers, or stacking cups.

→ Play Peekaboo and other imitating games.

→ Make funny faces in the mirror.

→ Bring baby outside to touch wet grass or leaves, hear birds chirping, and see the colors of nature.

→ Offer baby water play or let them explore outside with their hands (grabbing dirt, picking flowers, feeling rocks) with full supervision, of course.

Schedules During the Magic Window

Sample Feeding Schedule – 6 Months Old	
Expressed breast milk or formula: ~24 to 32 fl oz (720 to 960 mL) per day	
Solid food: Once per day when baby showing all signs of readiness	
6:30am	Bottle/Nurse
7:00am	Solid food
8:30am	Nap
10:00am	Bottle/Nurse
12:30pm	Bottle/Nurse
1:00pm	Nap
2:30pm	Bottle/Nurse
4:30pm	Catnap
5:15pm	Bottle/Nurse
5:45pm	Alternative time for solid food
6:30pm	Bottle/Nurse
7:00pm	Sleep (night feeds as desired)

This schedule is a sample. Know that it is okay if your baby's routine is different. Use this schedule as a starting point and adapt it in a way that works for you and baby. You can trust that your plan is working as long as baby is regularly peeing and pooping and baby is growing with themself as their own benchmark.

Between 6 and 8 months, baby's day likely follows a predictable routine. Some babies and families follow a set schedule, while others move through a rhythm for their day. Some babies sleep through the night at this age, and some continue to wake during the night for cuddles and feeding. Both are completely normal.

Baby is probably awake for 2 to 2½ hours at a time, and likely takes three naps per day, with some older babies beginning to transition to two naps. It's common for babies to have a shorter period awake before their first nap and a longer period awake before going to bed for the night, but not all babies follow this routine.

At first, we recommend offering solid food once a day as you get started. It's also okay if you want to skip a day here and there. During the Magic Window, you are working toward making one and eventually two meals into your baby's daily routine. As you begin, nurse or bottle-feed when baby is hungry and offer solid food at a time of day that works for you and baby. Aim to offer the meal 30 to 45 minutes after baby finishes breast milk or formula. This way, baby is likely to be happy, playful, rested, and ready to practice eating real food.

Oral Hygiene

Continue to practice oral hygiene, especially if baby's first tooth has popped. You can introduce a soft-bristled toothbrush or a soft cloth to gently brush baby's gums. Continue to focus on keeping this experience positive. If you have any concerns, discuss them with baby's dental provider at their first visit, which should be scheduled once that first tooth pops through.

Food and Nutrition During the Magic Window

This is the time to start solids, but it is not necessarily a period where baby eats much, if any, solids. Between 6 to 8 months of age, babies continue to get the majority of their nutrition and hydration needs met through breast milk or formula, and we do not expect any significant changes to how much breast milk and formula they drink this early on.

Many 6- to 8-month-old babies continue to nurse 8 or more times per day, with some nursing a bit less, and some still nursing during the night. If taking bottles, baby will typically take 24 to 32 ounces (720 to 960 mL)—sometimes more, sometimes less—of breast milk or formula (or a mix) across 6 to 8 feeds (or more) and still may take bottles during the night. Some babies may be down to 5 larger feeds, and this is just fine so long as they are thriving and growing well. Many babies may also be taking vitamin D drops as recommended by their care provider. For more on vitamin D and supplements, see Chapter 15.

This is incredibly important, so we want to repeat it: 6 to 8 months of age is a time for exploration and learning about eating real food; it is not typically a time for significant *consumption* of solid food. Some babies do figure out quite easily and quickly how to eat solid foods, especially pureed and soft foods, but many won't get it for a while. Many won't figure out real consumption until closer to 9 to 15 months of age. That said, don't get discouraged, as there are so many benefits to letting baby practice eating at this stage. For example, baby will benefit from being offered iron-rich foods and common allergens to help build their skills and familiarity with these important foods. With time and many opportunities to practice, how much solid food they eat will increase.

Water

Consider offering 2 to 4 fl oz (60 to 120 mL) of water per day from a cup or a straw for practice.

Baby's Progress at the Table

During the Magic Window, some babies simply learn to come to the table and explore the food with their hands. Others move from exploring to eating quite quickly. Both paths are normal. As long as baby continues to show an openness to coming to the table and a willingness to explore the food being placed in front of them in some capacity, they are progressing as expected.

Summary

✓ Most babies will show all the readiness signs to start solids around 6 months old and nearly all babies should begin exploring solid foods during the Magic Window.

✓ Focus on play that builds baby's core and shoulder strength to support their developing fine motor skills.

✓ Baby's breast- and bottle-feeding schedule likely will not change during this window, as solid foods are primarily for exploration and skill building from 6 to 8 months old.

✓ Six to 8 months of age is an excellent time to introduce your baby to teeth brushing if you haven't already. Even if baby hasn't cut a tooth yet, wiping their gums with a damp cloth after a meal can be the start of a toothbrushing routine.

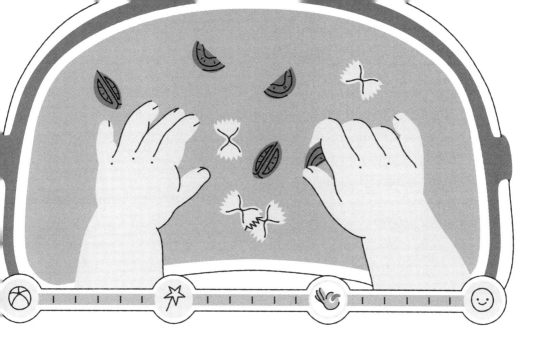

Chapter Eighteen

The Pickup Zone
(9 to 11 Months)

As baby approaches their first birthday, so many exciting things are happening. It's time for them to explore new food sizes and shapes, new skills, and some changes to meals at the table with you.[1] We call this baby's pickup zone for two reasons: first, this is the time that most babies figure out how to really use their fingers in a more precise way and feed smaller pieces of food to themselves they previously couldn't pick up on their own. Second, this is when the amount of solid food eaten at mealtimes often "picks up" for many babies.

Often, at this stage, babies progress from just exploring and spitting out food to chewing and actually eating more solid foods. Many are getting the hang of it by this time. For parents who have taken a more conservative approach, now is the time to move on from purees and spoons to finger foods. Even if baby is not quite ready to eat a greater amount of solid food, they are gaining new skills and showing improvements in how they hold, explore, and manage foods, which tells you they are on the right track. You can expect baby will be eating a greater variety of solid foods in larger quantities soon enough.

Use the following checklist to keep track of the things you can be doing with baby to support their development during this window.

Checklist

- ☐ Continue brushing baby's gums and any teeth.
- ☐ Introduce both small and big pieces of food.
- ☐ Progress to two to three meals each day.
- ☐ Think about babyproofing.
- ☐ Practice spitting out food or objects away from the table.
- ☐ Continue to offer a variety of foods, including iron-rich foods. Baby may have favorites or strong preferences, but try not to offer the same foods over and over.
- ☐ Continue to regularly offer common allergens, like peanut and egg.

Developmental Milestones

In the Pickup Zone, babies start to refine the use of their hands, and they progress from rolling and sitting up to scooting, crawling, standing, and potentially walking. As baby learns to move away from a trusted caregiver, separation anxiety and stranger awareness start to set in. There is a lot of variety of skill levels in 9- to 11-month-old babies, but all babies should be showing more interest in the world and in figuring out how to explore. Nine to 11 months of age is a time when gross motor skills provide an essential foundation for important fine motor skills, which support budding cognitive and communication skills, getting baby ready for some pretty huge developmental leaps.[2,3,4]

Gross Motor Skills

→ Sitting up independently
→ Crawling
→ Transitioning from lying down into sitting and from sitting to lying down
→ Pulling to stand up with support and cruising

During this time, baby goes from spending most of their time on their belly or back to being upright. Baby should be demonstrating more stable sitting balance without the need for supports, and most babies figure out how to transition from lying down into sitting up and safely back again. By 12 months of age, many babies start pulling to stand and cruising along while holding on to furniture or an adult hand. Some will take their first independent steps and others will be fully walking by 12 months of age. Independent walking is considered a 12- to 15-month-old skill, though, so no need to worry if your 9- to 11-month-old isn't there yet.

Fine Motor Skills

→ Using their thumb and first finger to pick things up
→ Learning how to point with their index finger
→ Turning pages in board books

Nine to 11 months is a time for babies to figure out how to use more refined hand and finger movements. During this period, most infants develop a pincer grasp—the ability to use their thumb and first finger together, separate from the rest of their fingers and palm, to pick up small objects—rather than using their whole hand to rake at items. This new pincer grasp is very much dependent on the new-found stability in baby's core muscles, which gives their shoulders and arms the stability needed to use refined fine motor skills. You should notice baby learning how to point and push big buttons with their index fingers as a step in developing the pincer grasp. Baby will pass objects between their hands, start turning the pages in board books, and manipulate objects more easily.

Cognitive/Language/Social-Emotional Skills

→ Pointing to communicate
→ Following simple directions
→ Saying their first word

The ability to experience the world upright and to point at things are game changers for learning and communicating. As baby starts seeing the world as you do, they learn they can show you what they are interested in by pointing at it. Pointing at items lays a foundation for baby to start to connect a name to different objects. At first, baby's receptive language is stronger than their expressive language. This means that baby understands words that you say but will not be able to say those words yet. For example, when you say, "Where's the doggy?" baby may be able to look around the room and lock eyes with your family pet, even if they cannot yet say "doggy."

That said, 9 to 11 months of age is a time when many infants say their first word. Babies are doing quite a bit of babbling at this age (dadadad, bagama). You may even hear baby pause or change their tone when babbling, almost as if they are having a conversation.

Some are able to use that babbling to consistently communicate a word with you. Sometimes parents do not realize the baby is using a word until much later because it's easy to assume baby is just babbling.

During this time most babies are becoming much more social, too. They are smiling, laughing, and showing affection by giving kisses, and they love to share their interest with you and look to see how you respond to something. Nine- to 11-month-olds are starting to understand object permanence, which means they know that when something leaves the room or is dropped, it does not disappear forever. They can anticipate that the item or person will come back. While separation anxiety definitely peaks in this period, baby is also learning that their trusted caregivers come back, too.

During this phase, baby is also playing around with the idea of cause and effect. They are little scientists who realize that they can affect the world around them, and their eager brains want to know "what will happen if I . . ." This phase can be frustrating as babies are driven to test cause and effect over and over again to see if the same effect happens each time or if something different eventually happens. In part because of their newfound object permanence (their understanding that objects still exist even if they are out of sight) and their interest in cause and effect, babies often love playing Peekaboo or other repetitive cause-and-effect games in this phase, such as filling up containers and then dumping them out, as well as throwing and dropping food.

Activities for 9- to 11-Month-Olds

Babies are really moving now, and their fine motor coordination is improving. Here are activities to build baby's overall strength and hand coordination for picking up smaller pieces of food.

Play Activities

→ Obstacle course: Use simple household items, such as pillows, tables, and chair legs, to make an obstacle course and encourage baby to crawl, scoot, or cruise around them.

→ Puzzles: Offer puzzles with knobs that baby can grab and turn over.

→ Tube play: Place small items in and through an empty toilet paper or paper towel tube.

→ Reciprocity games like the You're SO Big! game: You can initiate a back-and-forth with baby by saying, "How big is [name]? So . . . BIG!" and throwing your arms up in the air with the word "big." After doing this a few times, baby may "answer" you by throwing their hands up in response to "How big is [name]?"

→ Bubble time: Babies love to watch bubbles fly through the air, attempt to poke them, and even try to blow them themselves. This wet, sticky texture is great, especially for babies who are a bit more hesitant to touch foods such as yogurt, hummus, or other pureed or mashed textures.

Schedules During the Pickup Zone

Between 9 and 11 months there is a lot of variation in the typical schedule, as babies are adjusting to being awake for more of the day. During this phase, babies are often transitioning to two naps per day and slowly working their way toward three meals per day. Baby is likely awake for 2½ to 4 hours at a time, and most babies nap in the morning and in the early afternoon. It's common for babies to have a shorter time awake before their first nap and a longer time awake before bedtime, but this isn't the case for all babies.

Sample Feeding Schedule – 9 Months Old	
Expressed Breast Milk or Formula: ~24 to 32 fl oz (720 to 960 mL) per day	
Solid Food: Twice per day	
6:30am	Bottle/Nurse
7:00am	Solid food
8:30am	Bottle/Nurse (if desired)
9:00am	Nap
11:00am	Bottle/Nurse
12:00pm	Alternative time for solid food
2:00pm	Bottle/Nurse
2:30pm	Nap
4:30pm	Bottle/Nurse
5:30pm	Alternative time for solid food
6:30pm	Bottle/Nurse
7:00pm	Sleep (night feeds as desired)

This schedule is a sample. Know that it is okay if your baby's routine is different. Use this schedule as a starting point and adapt it in a way that works for you and baby. You can trust that your plan is working as long as baby is regularly peeing and pooping and baby is growing with themself as their own benchmark.

In terms of scheduling solid food meals, 9 months is a common time when families transition to two meals a day (if they haven't already), getting ready for three meals a day by 1 year. Nine to 11 months is a great time to work toward more consistency to help baby anticipate the typical time of day that they come to the table. It's still totally okay to skip a meal here or there, especially if baby is teething, sick, or overly cranky, as bottle and breast feeds are still prominent in the diet. Spacing solid food meals from breast or bottle feeds is a great goal during this time, as it will help baby come to the table a bit hungrier and more driven to explore the meal.

Oral Hygiene

For most infants, the first tooth emerges by 9 to 11 months of age, and the dental community recommends that you begin brushing baby's teeth as soon as they emerge. (Tooth eruption is quite varied, and it is normal if baby does not get teeth in the first year.) This is also a great time to establish primary dental care to familiarize your child with the dentist. Some dentists prefer to wait until your child is a bit older, but many are happy to see infants with their very first tooth.

That first tooth does not require toothpaste or even a toothbrush. You can wipe baby's teeth after meals and before sleep with a clean, soft washcloth, though an infant toothbrush dipped in water is also a great idea to begin familiarizing baby with this practice. If you prefer to use toothpaste, it's perfectly safe to use a tiny smear (about the size of a grain of rice) of toothpaste on a soft-bristled toothbrush, even though baby will very likely swallow this and not spit it out yet. If you have any concerns, discuss them with baby's dental provider at their first visit, which should be scheduled once that first tooth pops through.

Food and Nutrition During the Pickup Zone

Many 9- to 11-month-olds nurse 6 to 8 times per day, with great variability among babies in the number of nursing sessions. It's not uncommon for babies to still nurse during the night. If taking bottles, many babies will continue to take 24 to 32 ounces (720 to 960 mL) of breast milk or formula (or a mix) across 4 to 5 feeds (or more) and still may take a bottle during the night, but many do not bottle-feed at night anymore. You may notice baby taking in less breast milk or formula. Many babies may also be taking vitamin D drops as recommended by their care provider, and some also take an iron supplement. For more on vitamin D and supplements, see Chapter 15.

During this time, some babies naturally begin the process of cutting back on their breast and bottle feeds as they eat more solid foods at mealtimes. You'll find that bottles are not being finished, or are being refused altogether, or baby is nursing for shorter periods of time. This is expected, and nothing to worry about as long as baby continues to be active and engaged when awake, is overall content, and continues to make several wet diapers per day. If you have any concerns, please reach out to their healthcare provider.

Try to follow baby's lead—if they are consistently refusing to bottle- or breastfeed at a specific time, try going straight to solid food the next day. You may find that they request a breast milk or formula feed at a different time, and this is okay, too. Now is the time for trial and error, experimenting while slowly and gently guiding baby toward more solids and less breast milk and formula.

At the same time, if baby is not showing any signs of decreasing their breast or bottle feeds, that's completely okay. What matters most now is that baby is continuing to explore solid food and building chewing skills. While some babies do need a bit of a nudge from hunger to be motivated to eat more at the table, this can be accomplished in many situations by timing your feeds a little bit, and cutting back breast milk or formula feeds may not be necessary. You may try waiting 45 minutes to 1 hour between nursing or bottle feeds and solid foods, and up to 90 minutes to 2 hours as baby approaches the first birthday. Continue to offer baby a variety of foods, particularly iron-rich foods such as meat, poultry, seafood, beans, nuts, and seeds, which help meet baby's increasing iron needs at this developmental stage. Also, continue to regularly offer common allergens to help maintain exposures and sustain tolerance.

Water

Continue to offer baby 2 to 4 fl oz (60 to 120 mL) of water per day from a cup or a straw for practice.

Baby's Progress at the Table

Baby has had the opportunity to touch, taste, and explore a wide variety of foods by now, and we want to keep this momentum going. We know that the greater the variety of foods a baby is exposed to, the more likely they will be to accept a new one when you introduce it. Continue to work toward introducing common allergens, and if baby has not had a reaction, continue to offer these common allergens to baby regularly during the Pickup Zone.

This is also a great time to truly transition to sharing meals (if you haven't already). Baby is picking up on habits, routines, and the family's mealtime environment. Helping them see and get used to the idea of one meal for all is helpful now, as the toddler period is right around the corner. Remember—if baby does not eat or engage with the meal you offer, do not give them a different meal. (You are not a short-order cook.) You can offer a breast or bottle feed a bit after the meal (but not right after, as this can reinforce refusal), but start the habit *now* of not chasing baby's preferences. For more on refusal, see page 301 in the Problem Solving section.

Babies Need Practice to Learn to Chew

While some babies are able to eat enough pureed and mashed foods to fill the belly by 9 to 10 months of age, we want baby to learn how to chew more challenging textures. It is often much more challenging for baby to learn to chew than to learn to eat purees, and learning to chew typically involves a lot of spitting out. As they practice chewing, know that there is the safety net of breast milk or formula to help fill baby's belly. Allowing baby to self-wean off breast or bottle feeds as they fill up on purees can get you into a difficult spot where baby is stuck on purees. For more tips on this transition, check out Chapter 13.

Around this time, you will likely begin to see baby eating a greater quantity of solid foods. Around 9 months of age, the pincer grasp allows baby to pick up smaller pieces of food and get them to their mouth. As baby begins to figure out how to move these smaller pieces around in the mouth, don't be concerned if you see spitting and gagging again; it's completely normal. Continue to offer big pieces of food, which will help baby work on biting, tearing, and activating the senses in the mouth.

Remember, all babies need several months of low-pressure opportunities to explore food in this way, while watching a parent or trusted caregiver eat and enjoy food at the same time. If baby is happily exploring solids in their mouth at each meal but swallowing very little at 9 to 11 months of age, this is nothing to worry about. Be sure you are serving a variety of food textures, including soups, dips, sauces, and other naturally pureed foods that tend to be more easily swallowed, to help baby understand that food at the table can fill the belly.

For more information on common problems you may encounter, like spitting, throwing, pocketing, food refusal, and more, see the Problem Solving section in the back of the book.

Summary

✓ Around 9 months old, most babies start to develop a pincer grasp, which allows them to pick up smaller, bite-size pieces of food.

✓ Once baby has a pincer grasp, serve bite-size pieces of food or continue to serve larger pieces of food.

✓ Focus on fine motor activities that help baby refine their pincer grasp to help increase self-feeding efficiency at the table.

✓ For babies that have been eating only purees, this is an important time to progress to finger foods and foods with more variety in texture.

✓ For babies who have been introduced to a wide variety of food textures since 6 months old, you may see an increase in the amount of solid foods consumed during the pick-up window and a gradual drop in breast- and bottle-feeding.

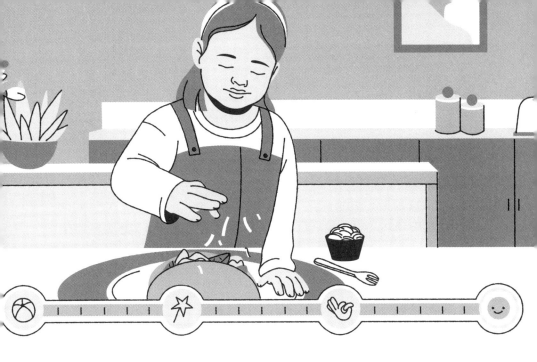

Chapter Nineteen

The Me, Me, Me Phase (12 to 18 Months)

Toddler land is wild. Every child is different, yet many common developmental and behavioral themes occur in the toddler years that make feeding and mealtimes a bit more complex. This phase is a time for putting boundaries and strategies in place that support your toddler's incredible brain development and autonomy while helping them through typical toddler challenges at the table.[1]

Weaning from formula and breast milk can be different journeys, so read the sections that are in line with your lifestyle and choices and get ready for the show.

During this transition, it's common for babies to figure out a certain movement or skill, and stop doing it for a period of time, but come back to it at the next meal. This is normal. Remember, babies develop on their own timeline, and there is a range of normal for when these skills emerge. If you ever feel concerned about your child's development, bring it up with their healthcare provider.

Use the following checklist to keep track of the things you can be doing with baby to support their development during this window.

Checklist

- ☐ If offering bottles, begin the transition to cups.
- ☐ If offering breast milk, consider your weaning plan.
- ☐ Look into toddler seating options if needed.
- ☐ Offer three meals a day (with two snacks if desired).
- ☐ Continue to serve a variety of flavors and textures.
- ☐ Continue to regularly offer common allergens, like peanut.
- ☐ Brush your child's gums and teeth each morning and night.
- ☐ Prepare for food refusal and toddler tantrums.

. . . And Solid Food Takes the Lead

This is a time where solid foods are meant to move from a supporting role to the star of the show, with breast or bottle feeds now becoming secondary to solid foods or weaned out entirely. This change can be smooth for some and full of confusion and anxiety for others. Additionally, growth starts to slow down a bit, which can lead to new fluctuations in appetite and can lead to food refusals. Toddlers are also entering a time of separation and independence, where they are driven to say "no," do the opposite of what we ask them to do, and insist on exploring and doing things their own way, on their own. In addition, toddlers have a much stronger memory and sense for what they like, meaning that they now have a stronger ability to remember that they do or do not like a certain food you served or that they want more of something you previously served.

Last, though definitely not least, between 15 and 18 months of age, most toddlers begin to show what researchers call "food neophobia," or a fear of new food. Whereas most infants are eager to explore any and all foods you put in front of them (they often put things we consider disgusting in their mouth when we aren't looking: sand, dog toys, dirty shoes, etc.), toddlers not so much. They approach new foods with less natural curiosity and more skepticism than infants, making it much more challenging to introduce them to new foods, or even familiar foods cooked or prepared in a new way. Bringing such foods into your meal if your child is not already eating them can be an uphill battle.

What adults would consider "bad behaviors" in toddlerhood are completely developmentally normal and will pass as your child develops more language to express themself and, eventually, the ability to work through feelings of disappointment, anger, frustration, and tiredness. They are not turning into "bad" kids or purposely trying to make things difficult (even though we know it feels that way!). They are managing a heavy load of brain development and cognitive change with still-emerging capacity. With that said, it doesn't make any of the behaviors easier to put up with, but they are completely normal and expected. We will share a preview of what to expect during this fun and challenging time and some basics of how to respond to these situations in order to keep your child safe and help them learn.

Developmental Milestones

During the Me, Me, Me Phase, baby is quickly becoming a full-fledged toddler. They are beginning to walk more often than crawl, and some are even running and climbing.[2,3] They are undergoing a massive amount of cognitive development during this window, deepening their understanding that they are unique individuals, separate from their trusted caregivers.[4,5] This newfound sense of self drives your toddler's desire to be independent and act contrary to whatever their caregivers suggest. This not only slows down getting out of the house (how long does it take your toddler to get the Velcro on their shoes closed on the way to daycare?) but also begins to play a part in mealtimes.

Gross Motor Skills

→ Standing without holding on
→ Walking
→ Learning to run and even climb
→ Challenging their balance

Twelve to 18 months of age is a time for movement. Most children learn to stand without holding on and walk between 12 and 15 months of age, and many will be fully walking, running, and even climbing by the end of this time. Your child is moving out into the world, and they are ready to explore.

Those first few steps will be wobbly, and we expect many falls as the child is gaining stability and balance. It takes time, often several months of repetitive practice, for your child to gain balance and confidence to navigate the world and all its different environments. Once your child is stable on their legs, they begin to explore further challenges with their balance, such as squatting down to pick up objects, then standing back up without holding on, and eventually lifting one leg to kick a ball. As with any other new skill, expect small setbacks as you go. A big fall might lead your child to want to be held more or to hold your hand while walking, even though they could easily do this independently the day before. This is normal. Go with it and know that as your child's confidence grows, they will need less and less support from you.

Fine Motor Skills

→ Picking up and manipulating small objects, like fitting wooden puzzle pieces with pegs back into the correct space
→ Scribbling with crayons
→ Feeding themselves with a spoon
→ Improved cup usage and control
→ Picking up smaller pieces of food and throwing things

All that newfound stability and strength in your child's core and legs, which allow them to walk and run, support the continued development of their fine motor skills. Toddlers begin to feel more stable through their core, which helps them to use those small muscles in the hands and fingers to do things like turning the pages of books, scribbling with a crayon or pencil, building with blocks, and feeding themselves with a spoon, with much more coordination and much less spillage than you might have seen at 6 to 12 months of age.

Speaking of fine motor skills for eating, your child will be able to pick up smaller pieces of food with more accuracy and efficiency. They will also get more accurate with throwing things they are not interested in (get ready for that). And 12 to 18 months of age is a time for your child to gain utensil skills, such as a spoon, a fork, and chopsticks, but don't expect much success just yet. If you have not already introduced these utensils to your child, now is the time. They will be messy, and they might resist or revert to using fingers quite frequently; this is part of the learning process and will fade out over time if you stay neutral, model how it's done, and continue to let your child practice.

Cognitive/Language/Social-Emotional Skills

→ Big leaps in problem solving and attention
→ Consistently strong opinions without flexibility
→ Big feelings, very little ability to self-regulate
→ A drive to be independent
→ An explosion in language

Your child's brain and social-emotional development is in high gear during the Me, Me, Me Phase. As they develop into their own person, they start to share interests, preferences, and opinions. Understanding that they can think and do differently than their parent can feel extremely exciting and completely overwhelming to some kids. As a young toddler's receptive language is strengthening, they can understand quite a bit of what you say to them, even if they are exposed to more than one language in the home, but their expressive language is still emerging. This means they may not have the words to describe how they are feeling or what they need, but they will still attempt to communicate those feelings and needs in some way, particularly as they gain a better understanding of what they like and don't like. Because of this, we expect some big feelings and some tantrums. Big feelings without the language to communicate those feelings leads to lots of crying and yelling.

Some families absolutely love this period, while others find it exasperating and confusing. Either way, this is a time for significant patience on your part. Your child wants to do it themself. They want to figure it out and their brain is hardwired to try. The more you are able to make space for this and allow your child to try, fail, try again, get frustrated, calm back down, and keep going, the more powerful learning will occur and the quicker your child will gain new skills.

Activities for 12- to 18-Month-Olds

Play in the Me, Me, Me Phase should follow your toddler's lead, but we'll give you some ideas that support mealtime development in a variety of ways.

→ Outside play: Time spent running, jumping, and climbing outside just before a meal can help prepare your child's body for eating by building hunger and expending energy before asking them to stay seated. Aim to have your toddler spend at least 15 minutes engaged in physical play prior to each meal.

→ Setting the table: Toddlers love to help, and having them help you set the table by sliding around chairs or carrying cups, plates, or silverware to the table can be an excellent form of gross motor play just before a meal. It's also completely appropriate to ask your young toddler to bring their plate to the sink after they finish eating.

→ Helping in the kitchen: Toddlers can help with pouring, tearing, washing, patting, stirring, pulling apart, shaking/mixing, and spreading. Washing fruits and vegetables, tearing lettuce, stirring a sauce, mashing cooked potatoes, and pouring ingredients into a bowl are all toddler appropriate.

→ Use descriptive words when talking about food such as "sour," "sweet," and "bitter" along with words such as "hot," "cold," "mushy," and "firm." Even describing simple things like the color of a food is a great way to engage your toddler at the table. Try to avoid words such as "yucky" and "gross," even when talking about nonfood items.

→ Grocery shopping with your child can introduce them to new foods and can challenge their ability to use their eyes to look around their environment, their language skills, and their memory. Ask them to help you find items on a shelf or join you in learning the names of items such as fruits and vegetables.

Schedules During the Me, Me, Me Phase

Sample Feeding Schedule – 12–18 Months Old	
Expressed Breast Milk or Formula: Anywhere from none to 14 to 20 fl oz (420 to 600 mL)	
Infant Formula: Up to 16 fl oz (480 mL) per day; 15 months+ typically none	
Solid Food: Three times per day + snacks	
6:30am	Wake-up
7:00am	Breakfast
9:00am	Bottle/Nurse (if desired)
9:30am	Nap
11:00am	Bottle/Nurse (if desired) or small snack
12:00pm	Lunch
2:00pm	Bottle/Nurse (if desired)
2:30pm	Nap
4:00pm	Snack
5:30pm	Dinner
7:00pm	Bottle/Nurse (if desired)
7:30pm	Sleep (night feeds as desired)

This schedule is a sample. Know that it is okay if your baby's routine is different. Use this schedule as a starting point and adapt it in a way that works for you and baby. You can trust that your plan is working as long as baby is regularly peeing and pooping and baby is growing with themself as their own benchmark.

Schedules vary greatly during this time, with some young toddlers taking longer naps than others, and some sleeping more hours overnight than others. Most young toddlers continue to take a morning and an afternoon nap, but it's not uncommon for some to consolidate and move toward one longer midday nap. Young toddlers tend to be awake for a max of 4 to 5 hours, with a shorter time awake in the morning and a longer time awake before bedtime, but this isn't the case for everyone. Bedtime may start to push a little bit later for some toddlers at this age. There is a big range of overnight sleep, with some young toddlers continuing to wake at night. Some young toddlers continue to nurse during the night, but this tends to be more for comfort than meeting a hunger need. If your young toddler is exploring solid food at mealtimes, practicing chewing, and swallowing food, no need to change your overnight schedule if it's working for you; but if your child is struggling to eat more solids, overnight feeds are a common culprit. Also, keep in mind that overnight feeds (both breast and bottle at this age) are associated with higher risk of dental cavities, but many families continue to offer feeds nonetheless, cleaning the teeth to the best of their abilities by wiping with a soft cloth after feeding.

During awake times, toddlers are busy and full of energy. You'll be fitting in three meals (breakfast, lunch, and dinner) as well as two snacks during the day. Some young toddlers who are still breastfeeding or taking bottles do so instead of snacks. Food tends to be offered every 2 to 3 hours during the day. There is no "typical" volume of breast milk or formula at this age, with some young toddlers taking zero and others continuing to feed. Keep in mind, many young toddlers can quickly and efficiently fill their belly with a breast or bottle feed. If your toddler is not interested in solid foods at mealtimes, consider how often they are nursing or bottle-feeding.

Oral Hygiene

It's important to engage your toddler in thorough oral/dental hygiene each morning and night, using a soft toothbrush and a grain-of-rice-size amount of toothpaste. While often impractical, cleaning the teeth after a nighttime feed is recommended, ideally with a gentle wipe, toothbrushing, or sip of water. While letting your toddler take the lead and try to brush their own teeth is an excellent way to get them interested and involved in the process, it's important for an adult to go through and thoroughly brush the teeth as well. The dental community also recommends flossing if any teeth are touching, or to use a floss pick to clean between the teeth. The American Dental Association recommends that you schedule your child's first dentist visit no later than their first birthday to help your child get comfortable with this healthy habit.

If your toddler resists toothbrushing:

1 Let them choose which brush they use.

2 Give control by letting them hold the brush.

3 Choose a flavor of toothpaste they are comfortable with.

4 Sing a song while brushing to help with length of time for brushing.

5 Brush in short intervals (3-2-1 break!).

6 Make it a game: I need to catch the tiger that is on your back teeth!

Food and Nutrition During the Me, Me, Me Phase

Weaning is often at the front of a parent's mind as their baby turns 12 months old. Should you wean? Do you have to wean? What if you or your child is not ready to wean; is that okay? Is it okay to stop breast milk or formula feeds right at 12 months of age if you're 100 percent ready? And if so, how do you feed your child? Lots of questions and lots of room for flexibility here.

The medical consensus is that most children can safely wean off breast milk or formula at 1 year of age. However, there are many reasons why some young toddlers aren't ready, and why parents may want to continue breast and bottle feeds. While the major governing bodies do recommend fully weaning from bottles by 15 to 18 months of age for oral and dental health and development, because of the health benefits for both the nursing parent and the baby, extended breastfeeding is supported as long as it's mutually desired by the child and parent.[6]

Skill building. Many babies are just not there yet. It is not uncommon or abnormal for a young toddler to still be building their chewing skills throughout the second year of life. Keep pressure at the table low while they continue to build these skills from 12 to 18 months of age and beyond.

Emotional value. Breast- and bottle-feeding both carry benefits beyond nutrition for infants and toddlers, with significant emotional and sentimental value for the parent and child that you may not be ready to part with.

Giving up the bottle and stopping or slowing nursing are very personal decisions. While there may be specific medical situations that mean you may have to wean at a certain time, in general, caregivers should not feel pressured to wean their baby before both baby and parent are ready.

Whatever your situation, 12-month-olds should be moving toward solid foods taking center stage, with breast milk or formula taking a supporting role. Even if you and your child are nowhere close to fully weaning yet, now is the time to actively guide the child away from primarily breast milk or formula and toward eating solid food at mealtimes. Breast- and bottle-feeding continue to have benefits through the second year of life, and at 12 months of age many children are just not capable of eating enough variety and quantity of solid foods to sustain their growth and development on solid foods alone.

Many parents believe that the goal is to swap out breast milk or formula for cow's milk or a milk alternative once the child is 12 months old. While this assumption that one can be replaced with the other is understandable, it is not recommended—and it can present new challenges in a toddler's transition to eating the food that you want to share at mealtime. The goal, when the child is ready, is to replace breast milk or formula with a wide variety of nourishing foods, with a beverage of water, cow's milk, or a calcium-fortified milk alternative served alongside each meal for hydration. Swapping out breast or bottle feeds for large amounts of cow's milk or a milk alternative may cause issues with iron deficiency, growth, development, and constipation; reduce the variety of foods consumed; contribute to food refusal and mealtime challenges; and negatively affect oral motor skill development. For more on cow's milk, see Chapter 15.

Water

After your child's first birthday, your toddler should aim to drink at least 8 fl oz (240 mL) of water per day. For some families this may feel like an impossible goal.

The best way to encourage water-drinking is to model drinking water in front of your child. To increase the amount of water your toddler drinks, ensure that water is easily accessible throughout the day outside of mealtimes. Other strategies include allowing your toddler to pour water with your help; adding ice, mint leaves, or pieces of fruit in a closed straw cup to add a pop of flavor or change in temperature; or having them choose a fun colorful cup.

For other children, water is easily accepted and enjoyed. While there is no official maximum amount of water a toddler is able to consume, most toddlers do not drink more than 30 fl oz (900 mL) per day. The amount of water a toddler drinks can vary day to day based on their thirst, which can be influenced by the foods they eat, their level of activity, illness, the weather, and many other factors. If you feel that your child is excessively thirsty, this can also be a sign of an underlying problem, and reaching out to your child's healthcare provider would be a good idea.

Baby's Progress at the Table

During the Me, Me, Me Phase, your child will make some nice gains in their oral motor skills. They will be biting into and tearing food with their front teeth, and you will likely see improved chewing skills, with the ability to break down and successfully swallow more resistive and crunchy foods. By 18 months of age, as chewing skills improve, you should feel that your child is capable of eating just about anything the other members of your family eat, with the exception of high-choking-risk foods. Because young toddlers are still easily distracted and very wiggly, we recommend you continue to modify or avoid those foods for a bit longer. For a list of high-risk foods, see Chapter 9.

This is also a time for your child to refine their eating skills, and a great time to start bringing utensils to the table if you haven't already and to do some focused utensil practice at meals or as part of playtime. Your child is likely ready to gain significant skill with utensils if you keep pressure low but give plenty of opportunities for practice.

You may also notice that your child uses their utensil at some meals but not at others; perhaps at dinnertime after a long day, they go back to using fingers. Using utensils is a complicated fine motor skill, and toddlers who struggle a little more with hand skills tend to favor eating with their fingers, leaning down to scoop food directly into their mouth or to lick food from the plate, or using their fingers to break large pieces of food apart. You may also see your child use their hands to scoop food onto a spoon or place it onto a fork as they are progressing.

The most helpful advice we can share about toddlers is to avoid serving separate meals from what the adults in the family are eating. Whenever possible, serve your toddler the same foods you enjoy. Eating with your toddler and sharing the same foods is a research-backed approach to increase the likelihood of your toddler eating the foods you eat and preventing normal toddler selectivity from turning into significant mealtime challenges and food refusals. Toddlers are social. When you serve special meals for your child or feed them separately from the rest of the family, they have lower motivation to stay seated, they are exposed to less variety of foods, and they tend to eat fewer fruits and vegetables. Sharing the same meals is hopefully a habit by now (you've been doing it for 6 months!), and maintaining this habit is critical to moving through toddler selectivity and keeping your toddler (and you) from falling into problematic mealtime routines.

Toddlers at the Table

It is in the wild universe of toddlerdom that you may begin to see some of the behaviors that many parents are afraid of—food throwing, food refusal, tantrums, and incessant requesting of snacks. This is *all normal* and has more to do with their brain development than the food you are serving. Several of the strategies used when your child was a baby will continue to be useful. For example, continuing to keep mealtimes pressure-free and offering variety. However, many 12- to 18-month-olds may need some new mealtime boundaries and strategies to be safe while eating and to avoid battles and picky eating.

Set a Schedule That Prioritizes Coming to the Table Hungry

Having a predictable (but flexible) schedule can do wonders in toddlerhood. Toddlers are very capable of recognizing patterns and respond quite well when they can anticipate what is coming next. Consistent mealtime schedules can even help your child's hunger hormones sync up to when you're eating, which helps them to intuitively prepare their brain and body to eat. While on-demand feeding is the norm in infancy, toddlers are much more capable of going longer stretches between meals, practicing patience, and getting on your meal schedule. One important benefit of a consistent but flexible schedule is that it provides times when the kitchen is closed. As your child learns that certain foods are favorites, they may start playing around with refusing to eat your meals, then requesting more preferred foods shortly after. Using a schedule makes it easier to reinforce your boundary because you know another meal will be coming in a few hours. This helps your child learn that new foods won't be coming immediately after one meal. Closing the kitchen between main meals and snacks can make the difference between a child who learns to eat what you serve and one who refuses, then cries for snacks 30 minutes later because they are still hungry. That said, there will be times when a child is still hungry, going through a growth spurt, catching up after illness, or experiencing something else that may disrupt and confuse their body's hunger and fullness signaling. It is entirely fine to be more flexible in these moments to support your child during these temporary seasons.

Intuitive eating, a style of eating that encourages honoring the body's natural hunger and fullness cues, often gets misconstrued as allowing your child to have free rein over all aspects of mealtimes. However, intuitive eating for children also encourages having flexible but predictable schedules; offering a variety of balanced meals with protein, fat, and carbohydrates to meet a child's nutritional needs and help them feel satisfied between meals; and allowing them to continue to self-regulate by deciding how much food to eat. Our job as parents and caregivers is to provide guidance and structure to help children thrive, while checking our emotions and making sure we don't make food a big deal.

It is also completely okay to provide a snack when requested, because your child may truly be hungry in between meals and is simply acting on their body's hunger cues. If the child ate their lunch, then requests a snack 30 minutes later, they are very likely hungry and it's a good idea to honor this. But if requests are in response to hunger due to food refusal at the meal, this can lead to more selective eating behaviors as your child knows they can refuse your meal and get a snack after.

If your 12- to 18-month-old is still nursing or taking a large amount of breast milk or formula and you see them throwing food, seeming disinterested in solids, refusing meals, or not staying seated in their high chair, these are clues that suggest they may actually need some support from you to gradually reduce milk feeds in support of eating more solid foods.

Setting some gentle boundaries around when the breast or bottle is available, stretching out time between milk feeds, or reducing the frequency or volume of breast or bottle feeds can help your child come to the table hungry and more interested in solids. This does not need to be full weaning. In fact, in these situations, it's best to start with small limits rather than dramatically cutting back on milk feeds in hopes that the child will start eating better at the table. You want to be certain that your child has the skills to eat a variety of foods before significantly reducing breast or bottle feeds.

Set a Rule: Food Stays at the Table

We know that children are at the highest risk for choking when they are moving—walking, crawling, or running—with food in their mouths. Setting a rule early on that food stays at the table or that your body must be seated if you are eating can save lives. Don't be afraid to physically pick your child up and hold them on your lap if they have food in their mouth—this is truly for their safety.

But we also know that most toddlers not only benefit from but need opportunities to move their bodies—and frequently. Sitting at a meal for more than a few minutes simply is too much to ask of many toddlers, and they can be much more successful with eating when they get breaks to move.

So we suggest the following: *food stays at the table but your body doesn't have to.* At mealtime, along with sitting, toddlers have the challenge of chewing and being exposed to familiar and new foods, the social aspect of mealtime, and hunger and the communication demand that comes with a meal. On top of this, an already wiggly toddler suddenly finds themselves feeling the need to do jumping jacks and run a marathon. So how can a caregiver keep their toddler safe while eating, while also meeting their movement need?

> **Food stays at the table, but your body doesn't have to.**

This rule allows a toddler the freedom to move when needed, while also maintaining the boundary that chewing and swallowing need to be done seated at a table for safety. Tips for keeping this rule in place:

1. **Let them sit and eat until they appear squirmy.** For some toddlers, this could be upward of 10 minutes, but for others, it may only be 3 to 5 minutes. When they appear antsy, explain: "It looks like your body needs to move. Let's take a break." Take them out of the chair and let them move in a safe, child-friendly area for 1 to 2 minutes. At the end of the movement period, explain, "Break is over, let's go back to the chair," and return them to the table and help them back into their seat/booster. You may even let them return on their own, without your guidance.

2. **Let hunger motivate them.** You may be concerned that they won't return to the table if they leave. This is where that hunger motivation comes in. When you follow a consistent schedule, your child will be hungry at mealtimes and more

likely to either stay seated or come back to eat when you give them space to roam but hold firm on that boundary that food cannot go with them. Additionally, toddlers are often motivated to return to the table because *you* are still at the table. They are social creatures, and they want to be near you. So, if you are seated, finishing your meal, they will likely come back.

3 **Make the nontable environment less attractive.** Lastly, you can increase the odds that your child will remain at the table by making the environment away from the table less attractive. Put toys away; allow your child to access only a small, babyproofed area with a few books or low-interest toys. Turn off screens and put away highly preferred toys for now, until you have finished your meal. You want the space away from the table to feel boring enough that your child notices their hunger and prefers to come back to see you and eat more food. If they still do not come back, this is the time to end the meal. While that can feel uncomfortable, remember that if you think they didn't get enough but you are following a consistent mealtime schedule, you all will be returning to the table in a few hours for another meal, which they will be more likely to eat because they are extra hungry.

Focus on Family Preferences, Not Just the Child's

Toddlers can be very demanding and quite clear about what they like and do not like. Unfortunately, those preferences are often based less on experience or true understanding and more on assumptions, so catering to their often-fleeting preferences or chasing your toddler's list of "will-eat" foods is not recommended. It nearly always results in an ever-narrowing list of accepted foods and prevents your child from doing the very important work of continuing to expand their flavor palate, food interests, and oral motor skills, all of which are an essential part of the early toddler years. Serving family foods and weaving a wide variety of foods into your daily and weekly menus, in addition to the foods you know your toddler enjoys, is an essential step in decreasing the likelihood of mealtime battles later on and growing your child's eating skills.

If your toddler has underlying medical, developmental, or sensory differences, more flexibility will be needed, and working with a medical team to provide individualized recommendations can be helpful.

Serve Options at Each Meal

Have we mentioned that toddlers have big opinions about nearly everything? One hack that can go a long way toward avoiding a battle and encouraging participation from your toddler is serving a few options at every meal. No need to go overboard with this, but having two to four choices (a main and a few sides, for example) at a meal gives even the more stubborn toddler some space to make their own choices and be in charge of what they eat at that meal, without you having to go back to the kitchen to find something new or sit through an epic meltdown.

Avoid Substitutions or Short-Order Cooking

Along those same lines, bringing a substitution to the table when your child refuses to eat what you served or engaging in "short-order cooking," where you cook up whatever your child requests, will likely set you up for more food refusals and mealtime battles. Instead, set your menu using the strategy we just discussed (with options) and stick to it. If you start short-order cooking, toddlers will quickly realize that the menu is not firm and food refusal or tantruming will get them different food options. With that said, we are all flexible human beings, and sometimes there is no time or capacity to handle a food-refusal tantrum. Plan your meals accordingly, and if your toddler is having a particularly tough day, lean into foods you are more confident they will eat. But again, don't chase their wants if they still refuse these foods.

Focus on Exploration and Engagement

Even if you use every one of these strategies, refusals and "yucks!" will happen. It can be extremely tempting to pressure your child to "try it" or "just take one bite" or even to promise a treat in exchange for tasting a nonpreferred food. These strategies can backfire, and research shows that they tend to make refusals worse. The goal is to teach your child the skill of tasting new food—being brave and curious and taking a chance. As we've discussed at length, skill development happens when a child is engaged and interested in the task and it's just the right amount of challenge. Forcing, bribing, or coercing the child to taste something may get one bite in the short term, but it will not develop that skill.

This does not mean you are helpless in the face of a refusal. Instead of trying to get your child to taste or eat the food, focus instead on exploring the food or engaging with the food in some way. Will they touch it? Look at it? Answer a question about it? Serve it to you? Dip it into something else or sprinkle a new seasoning or spice onto it? Will they be silly with it? Will they count it? There are so many ways for a child to explore and engage with food, and even though many seem like pure play, these strategies work to encourage eating without ever having to say "Taste it" or "Take a bite."

Why does this work? In part because play, exploration, and discovery lower a child's resistance to that food and put the child in a curious, positive mood, which makes them more receptive to it. If they happen to be hungry at the same time, the child often decides that tasting the food makes sense once they are more open to it. Also, these types of activities increase the child's familiarity with that food and make the food seem less scary, more approachable, and familiar. Remember that food neophobia we talked about earlier? When food becomes familiar, it starts to quiet the neophobia that tells your toddler not to eat it.

Get Comfortable Setting Boundaries

Parenting toddlers is a delicate balance of allowing independence and exploration while setting boundaries to keep your toddler safe and on task. Holding boundaries is not about something your toddler does but something *you* do. If your child does not respond to your request, you hold the boundary. Here are some examples:

> "It looks like you're having a hard time leaving the park. *I am going to* help you by picking you up."

> "Looks like you're having a hard time using nice hands with your brother. *I am going to* move you to this side of the room."

When it comes to boundaries around eating and meals, things can get a bit uncomfortable. The idea of setting a boundary around what behavior is appropriate for a meal and knowing that the natural consequence of that boundary being pushed is hunger later can be challenging for a parent. The research on toddler behavior shows that toddlers learn best when consequences are directly related to the choice they made or behavior they exhibited. In the case of a meal, the behavior or choice may be to throw food—and the natural consequence is that the food is now gone or not available. Will that lead to hunger? Likely. And you as the parent can help them navigate that discomfort. But this hunger reinforces the fact that thrown food is gone, and the child is able to recognize that they don't like the natural consequence that comes of that.

Boundaries that keep a child safe can seem easy (no, I won't let you play with scissors or run in the street), but holding boundaries that lead to a child feeling hungry can feel scary. Think about what limits feel appropriate to you, because this will come up a lot in toddlerhood. Some children will need more help than others with tuning in to hunger, fullness, and focus at mealtimes, and they may need a bit more trial and error with gentle guidance to figure this out.

Your Child Can Do This and So Can You

Mealtime is a common time for big opinions, overwhelming emotions, and boundary testing. A whole new set of mealtime strategies may be needed now that you've entered toddler land, and we're here to support you as things change. The strong foundation you laid in infancy matters. Along with the work you will put in during toddlerhood, this will set them up to be capable of safely eating a wide variety of foods. Playing the long game will carry your child into their school years and beyond as they grow into human beings who are equipped to make their own well-informed choices about which foods to eat and what their body needs to thrive.

Summary

✓ Around 12 to 18 months old solid foods will take on a more significant role in baby's nutrition, while breast and bottle feedings begin to take a supportive role or may be weaned out entirely.

✓ For baby, this is a time for movement and cognitive development and big feelings without the language to communicate those feelings. Baby also develops the feeling that they are unique individuals, wanting to do things their own way, which begins to play a part in mealtimes. This is a time for significant patience on your part.

✓ Toddlers can pick up smaller pieces of food with more accuracy. Twelve to 18 months of age is the time for your child to gain skill with utensils, such as a spoon, a fork, and chopsticks. Yes, it will be messy! That's part of learning. Let them practice.

✓ Fine motor skills: let them help you in the kitchen. Twelve- to 18-month-olds love to pour, tear, wash, stir, mix, and more.

Conclusion

As you close this book and begin the journey of bringing baby to the table with you, remember that introducing solids is not just about feeding—it's about connecting, sharing joy, exploring, and learning. It is a slow process, but you are laying the foundation for lifelong habits that extend far beyond the dinner table. The skills learned and practiced at every meal—patience, problem-solving, compromise, curiosity—are used in every aspect of life. You are fostering your child's relationship with food, one that is positive and full of discovery, but also their relationship to you.

Know that there will be many ups and downs. You will have bad days, and baby will have their own challenging moments. Missteps are a part of learning. Yet every meal is an opportunity to try again, to do it differently. On short-game days, when you are just barely getting by, allow yourself compassion. Know that you can always get back to your long-game goals tomorrow. In fact, making mistakes can strengthen adaptability, so when possible, celebrate those moments as opportunities to learn. The messiest moments are often the most powerful catalysts of growth.

If you take just one thing from this book, we hope it's the belief that you and your baby are both capable. Your baby is capable of learning these complex yet innate skills of eating the foods you serve, and you are capable of teaching baby to love mealtimes, and to trust and nourish themselves. Feeding baby should feel like a conversation, where you are both participants. Follow baby's lead but know that you will also guide baby on this journey. From the first bite through the challenging toddler years, every meal can be a unique opportunity to help them discover who they are and what they love. And our team will be with you every step of the way, guiding you. Lean on this book and the Solid Starts App to fill in the details, then jump in with joy.

Problem Solving

Here are our best tips for managing and working through the very typical yet hard and frustrating parts of starting solids. While in many circumstances it's a caregiver's job to simply back up and let baby try, other times there are some simple tricks for holding baby's hand a bit while they build their eating skills.

Overstuffing

While uncomfortable to watch, overstuffing is a part of the learning process as baby's brain begins to understand how much food should go in the mouth. Putting lots of food in the mouth sends a strong message to the brain of where there is and isn't space. Since baby can't look at the inside of their mouth, they rely on touch and feedback from the muscles in the mouth. This helps create what's known as a "map" of the mouth. So when baby stuffs too much food in their mouth, they get a clear picture of what's happening in there. Here's what you can do in the moment:

1 Stay calm. While it may feel like an emergency, it is not.

2 Calmly tell them, "That's too much; let's spit it out."

3 Clear food from the tray so baby does not continue to put more food in their mouth.

4 Gently lean baby forward so gravity can help them spit out the food. If baby pushes back, kneel down in front of them to encourage baby to look down.

It can be tempting to try to prevent overstuffing by putting one bite at a time on baby's tray. However, baby will still likely go through a phase of overstuffing once you stop limiting the amount of food on the tray, and the act of overstuffing does in itself help to end the problem once baby is more aware of the space in their mouth.

Food Is Stuck to the Roof of Baby's Mouth

Offer a dry, empty spoon for baby to suck on. The sucking motion can help dislodge the food and allow baby to either try to chew it or spit it out. You can also offer a small sip of water from a straw.

Food Stays in the Mouth (Pocketing)

Pocketing will happen as baby learns to move food around the mouth, but if it's happening often it can be a sign that baby is having a hard time moving the tongue side to side, or they need more touch input to recognize where food is in their mouth.

Here's what to do in the moment if baby is keeping food in their mouth:

1 Remind baby to swallow. You can show "swallow" by swallowing a bit of your own food (or drink) while running your hand from your lips along your throat and down to your stomach.

2 Coach baby. Tell baby, "You can spit that out," and exaggeratedly show how to spit out a small bit of food, while holding your hand in front of baby's mouth.

3 Offer a drink. If coaching doesn't work, offer a small sip of water, breast milk, or formula to drink, ideally, from an open cup.

4 Offer an empty spoon for baby to suck on. Sometimes this will give just enough of a cue to remind them to clear their mouth.

5 As a last resort, help baby lean forward (so gravity is on your side) and kneel so baby looks down at you.

How to Address Overstuffing and Pocketing

1 Build awareness: Unbreakable food teethers are excellent for this. Gnawing or sucking on these foods builds strength and coordination in baby's jaw and tongue muscles, while also giving lots of sensory input to the jaw, gums, tongue, and roof of the mouth. This helps build that mental "map" of the mouth.

2 Pump up the flavor! Offer baby lots of foods with slightly tart or sour bright flavors: oranges or lemons, mashed blackberries, marinara sauce, and tangy yogurt are all examples. These types of foods "wake up" the muscles of the mouth.

3 Brushing baby's gums, teeth, and tongue twice a day also "wakes up" and helps to "map" the mouth.

4 Let them investigate. Once baby spits out the wad of food, don't take it away! It may seem gross, but allowing baby to look at it, touch it, and even pick it back up and try again can be extremely valuable learning.

5 Go big! While it may seem contradictory, smaller pieces of food tend to get overstuffed and pocketed more. Try big pieces of food that require biting and tearing and slices too big for the mouth.

Swallowing Food Whole

This is common and not inherently unsafe. Baby is likely able to manage it, though it's not uncommon for baby to look a little pan-icked as the larger piece makes its way down the esophagus. Remember that there are two tubes: a food tube for eating in the back of the throat and a breathing tube in the front. The food tube is very elastic and made of muscle that pushes food down. The breathing tube is much more rigid, so if a large piece of food is swallowed in the food tube, it shouldn't stop baby from breathing through the breathing tube.

You can help baby work on chewing a bit more to increase their ability to break food down by offering unbreakable food teethers such as rib bones, chicken drumsticks, corn on the cob, mango pit, or cucumber spears. These trigger the chewing reflexes and help baby map the mouth. If baby's tendency to swallow food whole doesn't improve within a month or so, it's reasonable to seek additional support from a feeding therapist.

Gagging, Coughing, and Even Throwing Up

We've talked in detail about gagging and coughing and how both are normal protective responses as babies learn to eat and make mistakes along the way. Sometimes a very intense gag may even lead to throwing up—and in many cases this is completely normal. Try spacing out your milk feed and solid food meals by at least an hour so baby's belly is less full when they get to the table, and avoid sticky foods such as banana and avocado, fruits and vegetables with skins, and foods that scatter in the mouth, such as rice, which are notorious for causing intense gagging. Unbreakable food teethers are also excellent for babies with strong gag reflexes, as the deep touch and pressure sensation in the mouth helps to lessen the gag.

It's hard to know what's normal when it comes to gagging. Some babies are very gaggy while others gag much less. All of this can be normal but may also be a sign of an underlying medical issue like reflux or sensory sensitivities. If baby continues to gag at most meals after an initial learning period (one to two months of finger foods); is frequently becoming upset after gagging (crying, vomiting); gags at the sight of food; gags on most textures; or is vomiting at most meals, even on an empty stomach, it's worth discussing this with their healthcare provider.

Dropping and/or Throwing Food

Dropping and/or throwing food is simply an exploration of cause and effect. It can be a sign that the baby is "all done" or not hungry, or that the food is slippery or hard to pick up. Infants are also learning cause and effect, and dropping or throwing food is an exciting way to see what happens. If baby isn't hungry, end the meal. If the food is too slippery, hand food over to baby. If baby seems to be playing with cause and effect, ignore it at first. Tell baby, "Food is all gone!" and end the meal. Baby can have a bottle or breastfeed a bit later when they are hungry.

If You Want to Address It More Directly

1 Leave the food on the floor for a minute. Let baby realize that when they drop food, it goes away (cause and effect).

2 Pick up the food and replace it, saying, "Food belongs on the table."

3 Replace fallen food one or two times only.

4 End the meal. Remember, you can support baby's hunger with breast milk or formula. Ending the meal helps baby learn that throwing = my food goes away.

Some babies need to be shown *and* told. Stand next to baby and gently "catch" their arm as it shoots to the side to drop the food and coach them to bring the food back to the plate, saying, "Food belongs on the table." If baby is throwing to communicate that they are "all done," use the "catch" strategy and ask, "All done?" while signing, "All done." Replace the food on the plate and remove it swiftly. Repeat this each time it happens.

Some families like to use a "no thank you" plate or bowl, which can be a different color or shape to bring attention to it. This can be a place for your child to deposit food they do not want to explore instead of throwing it, but this concept likely won't "click" until toddlerhood.

Baby Hates Getting Cleaned Up

Because mealtimes are such messy endeavors and cleanup can be really upsetting for babies, we recommend waiting on the cleanup until the end of the meal and completing the cleanup away from the table. Bring baby directly to the sink, and allow them to play in water as you wipe their body, hands, and face. You can also offer them their own towel and guide them in wiping their own hands and face. A bowl or pitcher of water can also be fun for baby to dip their hands and clean up somewhat independently.

Baby Hates Having Their Hands Dirty and Won't Touch Messy Foods

Some babies are particularly sensitive to touching wet or messy textures and want food wiped off quickly if their hands or face become messy. If you notice this, try bringing a damp, soft cloth to the table and keeping it near baby at each meal. Show them that they can help you wipe their hands on this cloth whenever they become upset. If you are helping to clean them up, use a soft, damp cloth and warn baby first by saying, "I'm wiping your face on the count of three." Then count to prepare them and complete the wipe gently and as quickly as possible. Pairing a fun song with this can also help to decrease any discomfort as you wipe their face.

If baby refuses to touch messy textures at all, you can try preloading spoons for baby at first. You can also work on increasing their tolerance of messy and wet textures through playtime away from the table. One of our favorite ways to do this is through outdoor play. Playing in a yard, garden, or park grabbing leaves, putting hands in grass or even dirt or mud (with close supervision, of course), or playing with water and water toys can be a valuable way to get baby more familiar with this type of sensory input.

If you are noticing that baby has a hard time with a variety of textures at and away from the table (washing hair, grass outdoors, baby-safe paint, etc.), mention this to their healthcare provider, as it can be a sign of sensory sensitivities.

Food Refusal

After exposure to meals with positive, no-pressure modeling, if baby isn't exploring solid food or refuses to bring food to their mouth, start by chasing the "why." Remember, a child's behavior is communication.

Common Reasons for Food Refusal

1 **Baby isn't ready for solids:** Young babies may not be developmentally ready to start solids. If baby is 4 to 5 months old, consider waiting another month or so; if baby is 6 months old, wait a week or two, which can give baby some extra time to put those skills together.

2 **Baby isn't sure what to do:** You may need to bring their attention to the food by tapping the tray or calling their name. You can pick the food up and hand it to them, or stand it upright in something sticky such as yogurt. Bringing baby to the table often and eating in front of them is key to learning what is expected when food is presented. You can exaggerate picking up your food and bringing it to your mouth, chew with your mouth open, mimic chewing motions with your hands, and point to your throat and then belly when you swallow. Don't expect baby to immediately mimic you (although they might!), but constantly modeling is key.

3 **Baby is sleepy:** Reconsider what time of day you are bringing baby to the table. You may need to move solid food meals to a time when baby is more awake and alert.

4 **Baby feels pressured to eat:** Babies are very sensitive to pressure—both positive and negative. If a baby has been encouraged, pushed, or forced to eat, they may resist putting food in their mouths. As hard as it may feel, this is baby's communication that they need some time and space to learn on their own. Reset the situation. Get away from the table. Bring baby to your lap or hold them on your hip while you snack in the kitchen and allow them to reach for the food if and when they are ready. Remove all expectations that they are going to eat anything and let them take the lead. Wait for them to engage without any encouragement from you.

5 **Baby is too hungry:** Baby can quickly get frustrated exploring food at the table if they are *too* hungry. Consider feeding baby a breast or bottle feed 30 minutes prior to solid food meals and then offering a breast or bottle feed again at the end of your solids meal if needed.

6 **Food is too challenging:** Babies may refuse food when it is too challenging for them to pick up and get to their mouth. If the food is too small or too slippery, consider modifying it to make it easier for baby to be successful.

7 **Baby is not feeling well or is teething:** It is very common for babies to completely lose interest in solid foods when they are not feeling well or teething. This is normal and nothing to be worried about. Sometimes a virus can linger a bit, so it's not uncommon for baby to take some time to get back on track. In addition, illness can negatively impact taste and smell. Use comfort measures when baby is teething, such as soothing baths, holding and rocking, or pacifiers outside of mealtimes. Consider offering cold food teethers, such as a mango pit directly from the refrigerator or a frozen celery stick, at the start of mealtimes to help soothe baby's gums. If needed, offer mashes or purees rather than finger foods to reduce pain or discomfort at the table. Continue coming to the table, but do not pressure or force baby. If needed, sit them on your lap rather than in their high chair (this alone can be soothing) and keep food ready for them, but do not encourage them to eat it. Simply eat your own food and let them watch you and join in if and when they feel ready.

8 **Baby is uncomfortable in the high chair:** If baby is leaning backward, is slumped to the side, or the tray table is too high, self-feeding will be extra challenging, exhausting, and frustrating.

9 **Baby has a medical condition or developmental delay:** Certain medical conditions can impact baby's interest in solid food, such as acid reflux, constipation, and allergies. Occasionally, infants refusing solid food or struggling with self-feeding or learning to chew may have developmental delays or sensory processing differences that make it more challenging to develop these new and complex skills. Speak with your child's medical provider or early intervention team for support.

If baby still doesn't seem to understand that food goes in the mouth, here are some things you can try. These strategies include the adult sharing the same piece of food with baby. We would be remiss not to mention that these practices potentially share oral bacteria between parent and baby. It's important for parents and caregivers to be aware of this if choosing to use these strategies.

1 Take a bite of the food and hand over that piece of food to baby.

2 Hold the food piece between your front teeth and lean in toward baby for them to take it from your mouth.

If you've tried all of these strategies and none of them are working, consider taking a two- to three-day break from solids. When you try again, do so away from the high chair for another two to three days. You can sit on a blanket in the living room or outside. Have baby sit on your lap or with another trusted caregiver. Changing the environment can make a significant difference.

If you see no interest at all after attempting these strategies, consider talking to your child's healthcare provider and requesting a referral to a feeding therapist for a more individualized evaluation.

Getting Back on Track After Illness/Teething

It is not uncommon for babies to refuse solid foods when they are sick, but also for a period of time after they have recovered. Continue to focus on breast and bottle feeds and maintain your typical mealtime routine. Bring baby to the table to participate in mealtime, but don't expect them to consume much of anything. With low-pressure exposure, baby will get back on track.

Constipation, Gas, Blowouts, and More

When starting solids we tend to focus on what occurs at the mouth—skill building, exploration, and consumption—yet a lot is occurring in baby's digestive tract as well! For one, their gut microbiome is maturing and diversifying, and this is the first time it has seen solids. For exclusively breastfed infants, the first change you might note is the smell and consistency of baby's poop. Poop color and even poop texture will begin to show more variation depending on what and how much baby has consumed. If you are ever concerned, snap a picture of poop and discuss it with your child's primary healthcare provider.

Pooping While Eating

Is baby pooping while seated at the table? We have a reflex in our bodies called the gastrocolic reflex that is triggered after meals. When food enters the stomach, a signal is sent to the brain that says, "Food is here!" and then the brain sends a signal down to the colon that says, "Make room!" In response, the colon squeezes, ultimately resulting in the urge to poop. Some babies have a very sensitive reflex, resulting in bowel movements during or immediately after meals or feeds. This is okay so long as they are growing well.

There is not much we can do (or should do) to stop a bowel movement from occurring. If baby does not want to return to the table following the diaper change, sometimes we try moving the meal to the floor, like a picnic, as a way to re-engage baby.

Crying but Poop Is Soft

Pooping requires two things to happen: you have to relax your pelvic floor while also increasing your intra-abdominal pressure (bearing down). Young infants (usually under 9 months) can have problems coordinating these two things and experience a condition called infantile dyschezia, a nonworrisome problem when an infant struggles to learn to push poop out. Typically, infants will cry for at least ten minutes and appear as if they are attempting to poop—straining, bearing down, crying. They may even turn red in the face before successfully passing a soft poop. Crying is baby's attempt to generate intra-abdominal pressure; they are not in pain. The body typically resolves this issue on its own with time and practice. Suppositories and rectal stimulation are not recommended.

Teething Poop?

Contrary to popular belief, teething is not strongly associated with diarrhea or mucus-like poop. The top five most common symptoms experienced with teething are gum irritation, irritability, drooling, sucking on fingers/toys, and loss of appetite. Certain liquid pain medicines contain ingredients that can soften poop, a reason why changes in poop may occur during teething. If baby is having several loose bowel movements per day, do not be quick to blame it on teething, and speak to their medical provider.

Gas

Gas is quite common after solid foods are introduced. The most common culprits are very fiber-rich foods, such as broccoli, asparagus, beans, legumes, and pitted fruits. If baby is experiencing gas or tummy discomfort, start with smaller quantities of these foods and gradually increase over time to allow baby's digestive system to adapt and adjust. Fiber is excellent for developing gut microbiome and supporting bowel movements. If gas is waking baby up at night, try temporarily reducing some of these fiber-rich foods until symptoms resolve, and then gradually add them back in. To help address gas, tummy time (physical activity in general), warm baths, bicycle kicks/ knees to chest, and abdominal massage may help. And when in doubt, don't hesitate to check in with baby's primary healthcare provider.

Blowouts

While blowouts are common during the first few months of life and during illnesses, they can also occur after solid foods are introduced. The common food culprits that cause blowouts are similar to those that can cause gas. We see blowouts when larger quantities of fruits, vegetables, and beans are ingested. Ensure that baby's diaper is the right size to help reduce the risk of leakages. Blowouts should improve with time as baby's digestive system becomes more accustomed to solid food. If blowouts are happening regularly, in the absence of any illness, be sure to check in with baby's primary healthcare provider.

Diarrhea or Watery Poop

Most often, loose, watery bowel movements occur in conjunction with a viral illness ("stomach bug") and will resolve with time. While the BRAT (bananas, rice, apple, toast) diet was once recommended to treat diarrhea, it is now outdated advice. There are no specific dietary restrictions for baby, though foods with high sugar and fat content can exacerbate diarrhea, so it is often recommended to temporarily minimize these foods during the illness. If baby is having very watery bowel movements, focus on keeping baby hydrated and looking for about four full wet diapers per day. Sometimes an oral rehydration solution (such as Pedialyte or DripDrop) is needed, but often breast milk or formula is enough. Plain water is not recommended for infants during times of illness. Sports drinks such as Gatorade or Powerade are inappropriate as they are high in sugar, which can make the diarrhea even worse. It is never recommended to give any medication to stop diarrhea. If diarrhea becomes bloody or is accompanied by vomiting, if baby is showing signs of dehydration (inability to make tears, dry chapped lips, little to no energy, few wet diapers), or if you have any other concerns, please consult with baby's pediatrician right away.

Mucus in Poop

The digestive tract's primary role is to digest food and absorb nutrients while also protecting the body from outside organisms and invaders. Our intestines are lined with a mucus layer that not only helps pass food and poop through the intestines but also serves as a line of defense against intruders. Small amounts of mucus in bowel movements are normal. Excessive amounts of mucus may be concerning, especially if accompanying other symptoms such as difficulty with weight gain, eczema, or infections. Cow's-milk protein allergy, for example, may lead to mucusy bowel movements without any evidence of blood or belly pain. If you have any concerns, please do not hesitate to talk with baby's pediatrician.

Undigested Food in Poop

It is common (and completely normal) to see partially digested bits of food in baby's poop! Solid food can pass quickly through a baby's digestive tract. The faster the food travels, the less time it has to be fully digested. Some food elements, especially fiber-rich foods, are harder for the body to break down. Some examples of what you may see in baby's diaper include the outer shell of corn kernels, the outer skin of beans, the skin of vegetables and fruits, and whole seeds. Juice and antibiotics can cause food to move rapidly through the intestines as well, leading to very loose poop with bits of food in it. Remember that baby is developing chewing skills at this age. This can also result in seeing pieces of carrots, broccoli, and blueberries, among others, in the poop. In general, as long as baby is comfortable and thriving, this is not worrisome. If you consistently see undigested food in baby's poop and baby is having difficulty gaining weight, we strongly suggest that you reach out to baby's pediatrician.

Is My Baby Constipated?

Constipation is quite common. Constipation-related concerns are responsible for at least 3 percent of all general pediatrician visits and at least 25 percent of all pediatric gastroenterology visits. Seventeen to 40 percent of kids who are constipated began having bouts of constipation starting in infancy.[1] Constipation is loosely defined as the passage of infrequent, hard, and sometimes large-diameter poop.[2] For example, if baby poops every three days but the poop is very soft, it is highly unlikely that they are constipated. Following the introduction of solids, we can see firmer, less frequent, or even looser bowel movements.

How Can Constipation Be Treated?

Before jumping to medications, you can usually address constipation by altering what is being offered to baby. If baby is consuming a lot of rice cereal or low-fiber foods, add some more fiber- and probiotic-rich foods such as avocado, pear, ground flaxseed, berries, yogurt, whole grains, and beans. For children older than 6 months, a few ounces of water per day (not to exceed 8 ounces per day) may also do the trick. Physical activity helps move poop along, so plenty of floor time may also be beneficial. Warm baths and abdominal massages may help as well. If, despite your best efforts, baby is still suffering from constipation and difficult bowel movements, or if you feel like you are eliminating foods from baby's diet to address the constipation, check in with baby's primary healthcare provider for further guidance and evaluation.

Pooping While Sleeping

Control over bladder and bowel function is gradually acquired over time, so pooping while sleeping is normal, especially if baby is feeding during the night. While we are asleep, our bodies and digestive system are relaxed, thus making it easier for bowel movements to pass. Looking at baby's current schedule, if at all possible, you may consider trying to lengthen the time between eating and going to bed (much easier said than done!). Additionally, you may consider giving baby a warm bath after dinner to help relax baby and maybe even facilitate a poop before bed.

Infant Reflux

Reflux or spitting up is very common in infants; it tends to peak at 4 months of age and disappear by 12 months of age, as baby's digestive anatomy becomes more mature.[3,4] Most babies are "happy spitters" in that they are completely unfazed by their reflux episodes and continue to eat and grow well without medication or medical intervention.

Historically, pediatricians recommended adding cereal to the bottle for reflux; however, the American Academy of Pediatrics (AAP) and the CDC now advise against this practice. Adding cereal to the bottle before baby is developmentally ready displaces nutrients and fluid baby would have normally consumed in breast milk or formula.

In some babies, it is thought that reflux may be associated with cow's-milk protein allergy (CMPA). Fortunately, most babies tend to grow out of this. If CMPA is a concern, reach out to your pediatrician for further support. Baby may need to be switched to a hypoallergenic or amino-acid-based formula. For breastfed babies, mom may need to start a diet free of dairy.

Tips for Reflux

→ Avoid overfeeding: try offering smaller feeds more frequently or spacing out feeds. Eating too much food at once may worsen reflux.

→ Optimize positioning after feedings: holding baby upright for 15 to 30 minutes after a feeding can help reduce the incidence of reflux.

→ Burp baby frequently during feeds: this can help reduce reflux by avoiding burping when the stomach is full.

→ Make sure the diaper isn't too tight: this may put too much pressure on the abdomen and lead to reflux.

→ If baby is formula-fed, talk to your pediatrician and pediatric dietitian about the options of formulas that are more reflux-friendly.

→ Consider the possibility of cow's-milk protein allergy if reflux is persistent and bothersome to baby.

→ Avoid exposure to tobacco smoke.

→ Babies with reflux may be more likely to throw up if and when they gag. Babies with reflux can benefit from spacing out milk feeds and solid food meals by 1 hour, even at the beginning of solids.

→ Get constipation under control: when constipation is an issue and not under control, it can contribute to reflux. Think of this like a plumbing issue: if things aren't flowing, there will be traffic jams.

A small percentage of babies have gastroesophageal reflux disease (GERD), which is when reflux causes complications such as irritation to the esophagus (eating tube), resulting in pain, asthma, or pneumonia. If you feel like your baby is suffering from GERD, please let their primary care physician know right away.

Signs Baby May Have GERD or Something Else

→ Arching the back or twisting the neck to one side as if in pain after a feed

→ Refusing to eat

→ Crying during feeds

→ Forceful or projectile vomiting

→ Spitting up blood

→ Coughing while feeding

→ Choking after refluxing

→ Difficulty gaining weight

→ Baby begins refluxing after 6 months of age

When to Get Help for Feeding Concerns

So many issues fall into the "it's normal" bucket when it comes to learning to eat that it's hard to know when to ask for more help. Anytime you have a question or concern, your pediatrician or pediatric healthcare provider is the first step. Sometimes a little reassurance is all you need. Here are some bigger challenges that warrant evaluation by your child's provider and potentially a referral for more help.

1 No interest whatsoever in food and eating, despite significant time, modeling, and pressure-free opportunities for exploration

2 Crying at the sight of the high chair or refusal to come to the table

3 Continued frequent gagging on most or all foods, especially if combined with vomiting

4 Refusal to touch any foods

5 Significant changes in weight, lack of weight gain, or difficulties with growth

6 Significant decreases in daily wet diapers

7 Overall lethargy or low energy

8 General inconsolable irritability

9 Hard, difficult-to-pass poop

10 Visible blood in poop

11 Frequent coughing and sputtering at most meals, especially if paired with frequent upper respiratory infections or unexplained fevers

12 Occasional choking incidents while baby is seated calmly in a supportive seat. Choking requiring intervention is quite rare. If you need to provide choking rescue more than once during this phase, further evaluation may be indicated.

If you are concerned, ask. Talk to your pediatrician about a referral to a pediatric feeding therapist, swallowing specialist, pediatric dietitian, or other pediatric medical specialist.

Further Resources

SolidStarts.com
Solid Starts App
Solid Starts PRO

Resources for Families with Allergies

We know firsthand how stressful and challenging life can be when a child has a food allergy. Fortunately, there are some incredible resources for parents and caregivers of children with food allergies. Here are just a few:

FARE (Food Allergy Research and Education)

FARE is the leading resource for food allergies in the United States. It's an excellent resource—a comprehensive website with support groups, detailed lists of foods to avoid if baby has a food allergy, and downloadable tools to post in your home.

National Institute of Allergy and Infectious Diseases

A leading research organization that seeks to understand, treat, and prevent allergic, immunologic, and infectious diseases.

American Academy of Allergy, Asthma & Immunology

A professional membership organization dedicated to advancing the knowledge and practice of allergy, asthma, and immunology for optimal patient care.

American College of Allergy, Asthma & Immunology

A medical association of allergist-immunologists and allied health professionals. Includes a tool to help you find an allergist near you.

Kids with Food Allergies

Part of the Asthma and Allergy Foundation of America. This website contains a terrific database of recipes that are allergen-free.

U.S. Centers for Disease Control and Prevention (CDC)

The CDC website includes a useful resource for managing allergies at school.

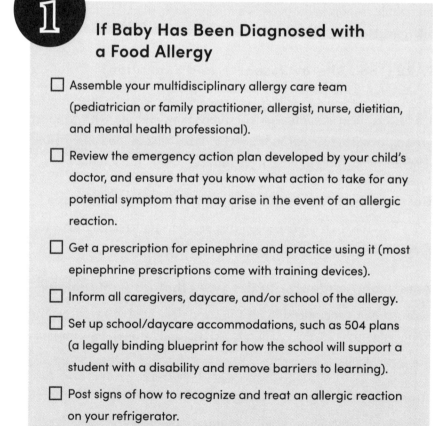

If Baby Has Been Diagnosed with a Food Allergy

- ☐ Assemble your multidisciplinary allergy care team (pediatrician or family practitioner, allergist, nurse, dietitian, and mental health professional).

- ☐ Review the emergency action plan developed by your child's doctor, and ensure that you know what action to take for any potential symptom that may arise in the event of an allergic reaction.

- ☐ Get a prescription for epinephrine and practice using it (most epinephrine prescriptions come with training devices).

- ☐ Inform all caregivers, daycare, and/or school of the allergy.

- ☐ Set up school/daycare accommodations, such as 504 plans (a legally binding blueprint for how the school will support a student with a disability and remove barriers to learning).

- ☐ Post signs of how to recognize and treat an allergic reaction on your refrigerator.

- ☐ Train all caregivers on what to do in the event of an allergic reaction.

☐ Take stock of your kitchen and pantry and read labels closely. Mark both the container and lid of foods containing allergens with "Do not serve to baby." Consider having separate cabinets to help make organizing and navigating the kitchen easier.

☐ Schedule regular follow-up visits to monitor for resolution of the allergy.

☐ For persistent food allergy, discuss treatment options (such as sublingual immunotherapy, oral immunotherapy, or biologics) with your allergist.

Epinephrine: Frequently Asked Questions

When it comes to epinephrine for the treatment of food allergy reactions, families often have a lot of questions. The following are some of the most common questions families ask.

Can you administer an epinephrine injection through clothing?
Yes, autoinjectable epinephrine can be administered through clothing.

Can you use an expired epinephrine injector?
Yes. Studies have demonstrated that when kept in a temperature-controlled environment, autoinjectable epinephrine can maintain significant efficacy for up to three years after the expiration date.[1,2,3] That said, only use an expired epinephrine device if you don't have access to one that is up to date. It is important that schools and daycares be given epinephrine autoinjectors that are up to date and not expired. School regulations don't allow them to accept expired pens.

Can you use epinephrine for FPIES?
Epinephrine does not treat the symptoms of FPIES. For a mild FPIES reaction that consists of one or two episodes of vomiting, oral antinausea

medications can be helpful. For a severe FPIES reaction that results in shock, the best treatment is IV fluid replacement and possibly steroids, depending on the patient.

Can you use an adult epinephrine injector on a child if necessary?

You have to be careful. The needle length on the adult EpiPen is longer than the one on the junior-strength device. On a very small child or baby, there is a risk that the longer needle might penetrate through the muscle and hit bone. That said, if it's a life-or-death emergency, it's better to use the adult pen than nothing at all. Administer the injector in the upper outer thigh, where the muscle looks and feels the thickest. Pinching the muscle between your thumb and pointer finger can lift the muscle up and reduce the risk of the needle impacting the femur bone.

How many epinephrine injectors do I need for a child with allergies?

Keep a minimum of two at all times. Make sure epinephrine is available at school/daycare, with babysitters, and anywhere else baby spends time. Keep expired pens as well, at least for a little while.

What do you do if there's a severe reaction and you do not have epinephrine?

Call 911, inform the operator that your child is experiencing a severe allergic reaction, and request an ambulance with epinephrine on board. While waiting for help to arrive, the operator will talk you through the steps to monitor and stabilize your child.

How do you know if a second dose of epinephrine is needed?

A second dose of epinephrine should be administered if symptoms of the allergic reaction are not improving within 3 to 5 minutes of the first dose (or if existing symptoms worsen or any new symptoms develop anytime after the initial injection/administration).

Emergency Resources

American Red Cross

Find child and baby CPR training classes and download the printable step-by-step guide.
www.redcross.org

American Heart Association

Check out the infant CPR training kit available for purchase.
https://cpr.heart.org

Solid Starts

Download our free infant rescue and toddler rescue guide.
SolidsStarts.com

Acknowledgments

This book was an incredible labor of love that required deep collaboration and commitment from many people.

First and foremost, we want to thank our families, particularly the kids in our lives who have humbled and inspired us from the moment they entered this world. This includes the children of so many parents and caregivers within the Solid Starts community who have shared their stories and experiences so others could learn. Each of you helped make Solid Starts what it is today, and we hope that one day in the future you will read this message and be proud. You have helped so many families learn, grow, and find joy at the table together: Aaïla, Aarav, Adie, Alex, Amália, Amaris, Amelia, Anjani, Aqeel, Asher, Ava, Beau, Benjamin, Bennett, Beth, Blythe, Bobbi, Broly, Caden, Callie, Calum, Charles, Charlie, Cleo, Cooper, Eduardo, Elena, Elisa, Elliott, Emerson, Emilia, Emilio, Eunoia, Eva, Evie, Gin, Gus, Hannah, Hannah Sierra, Hawii, Isar, Isla, Julian, Juliana, Juliet Rose, Kai, Kaia, Kalani, Laila, Leila, Lena, Leo, Lina, Logan, Louie, Lucy, Maëlys, Maeve, Mahalia, Malcolm, Malden, Marcella, Marshal, Max, Maya, Mika, Mila, Miles, Nico, Nkosi, Oliver, Olivia, Oscar, Owen, Patrick, Rafael, Raleigh, Riley H, Riley L, Río, Quaide, Quentin, Savannah, Sebastián, Sevigne, Sevy, Shehzad, Silas, Sofia, Theo, Tifa, Wei Wei, William, Yara, Zeke, and Zuri.

We owe a debt of gratitude to the entire Solid Starts team for their contributions to this book. In particular, we want to give a big hug and thanks to Kate Lindquist, our champion editorial leader, who has toiled behind the scenes to make this book move from the scrap of an idea to a reality. She helped shape its vision, charted the course and kept us on track, aligned our thinking along the way, checked us when we needed it, listened and calmed us when we were flustered, and shared her invaluable insight at every step. This book would not have been possible without her.

We are especially grateful to our feeding therapy team at Solid Starts, including Marisa Suarez, Alexia Derma Salazar, and Jenna Longbottom. Marisa and Alexia carried forward so many aspects of our day-to-day work at Solid Starts so that we had time and space to write this book, and Jenna's eagle eye made sure that every line of this manuscript was factually correct and grounded in the literature. Chelsea Synyahl-Gleisner, Katja Jylkka, Kelly Stange, and Nikki Silvestri were always by our side with wise feedback, suggestions, and support when we needed it.

Cait Hoyt, our agent at Creative Artists Agency, believed in this book from the moment we pitched the idea, and we are indebted to her for helping us find the best editors to bring it to life. We feel incredibly lucky to have worked alongside an incredible editorial team, particularly Libby Burton and Sandra Bark, who took what we wrote and made it better. From the very beginning, these amazing women embraced our vision and stayed by our side at every step of the way to help us realize it. We are particularly grateful for their abilities to turn complexity and chaos into compelling copy with logical narrative and simplicity in message.

We thank the creative minds of Carmen Deñó, Lucy Andersen, and T. M. Detwiler, who designed illustrations and infographics in this book. These artists faced one of the biggest challenges: using a two-color format to create works that feel like Solid Starts, which has relied heavily on photographs and videos in our digital storytelling to date. We are so impressed by their abilities, and we hope you love their work as much as we do.

While Solid Starts is often cited as a go-to source for infant feeding, we are certainly not the first (and we won't be the last!) to champion the idea that babies can practice eating real food as soon as they are ready to start solids. We thank the many infant feeding specialists, particularly Dr. Gill Rapley, and child development authorities, particularly Dr. Tina Payne Bryson, who came before us. These pediatric professionals have inspired our work in so many ways, and they have contributed to this book with their research, theories, expertise, and wisdom.

Notes

Introduction

1. Rapley, G., & Murkett, T. (2010). *Baby-led weaning: The essential guide to introducing solid foods—and helping your baby to grow up a happy and confident eater.* New York: The Experiment Publishing.

Chapter One

1. Brown, A., & Lee, M. (2010). Maternal control of child feeding during the weaning period: Differences between mothers following a baby-led or standard weaning approach. *Maternal Child Health, 15*(8), 1265–1271. doi:10.1007/s10995-010-0678-4.
2. Scaglioni, S., De Cosmi, V., Ciappolino, V., et al. (2018). Factors influencing children's eating behaviours. *Nutrients, 10*(6), 706.
3. Surette, V. A., Smith-Simpson, S., Fries, L. R., and Ross, C. F. (2022). Food texture experiences across age groups in 4- to 36-month-old children in the United States. *Journal of Texture Studies, 53*(1), 18–30.
4. Nicklaus, S. (2011). Children's acceptance of new foods at weaning. Role of practices of weaning and of food sensory properties. *Appetite, 57*(3), 812–815.

Chapter Two

1. Bentley, A. (2014). *Inventing baby food: Taste, health, and the industrialization of the American diet.* University of California Press.
2. da Costa, S. P., Remijn, L., Weenen, H., et al. (2017). Exposure to texture of foods for 8-month-old infants: Does the size of the pieces matter? *Journal of Texture Studies, 48*(6), 534–540. doi:10.1111/jtxs.12271.
3. Le Révérend, B. J., Edelson, L. R., and Loret, C. (2014). Anatomical, functional, physiological and behavioural aspects of the development of mastication in early childhood. *British Journal of Nutrition, 111*(3), 403–414. doi:10.1017/S0007114513002699.
4. Food Allergy Research & Education (FARE). (n.d.). *Learning early about peanut allergy (LEAP).* Retrieved April 17, 2024, from https://www.foodallergy.org/resources/learning-early-about-peanut-allergy-leap
5. Perkin, M. R., Logan, K., Marrs, T., et al., & EAT Study Team (2016). Enquiring About Tolerance (EAT) study: Feasibility of an early allergenic food

introduction regimen. *Journal of Allergy and Clinical Immunology, 137*(5), 1477–1486. doi.org/10.1016/j.jaci.2015.12.1322.

6. Natsume, O., Kabashima, S., Nakazato, J., et al. (2017). Two-step egg introduction for prevention of egg allergy in high-risk infants with eczema (PETIT): A randomised, double-blind, placebo-controlled trial. *Lancet, 389*(10066), 276–286. doi:10.1016/S0140-6736(16)31418-0.

7. Morris, Z. S., Wooding, S., and Grant, J. (2011). The answer is 17 years, what is the question: Understanding time lags in translational research. *Journal of the Royal Society of Medicine, 104*(12), 510–520. doi:10.1258/jrsm.2011.110180.

8. World Health Organization. (2011). *Exclusive breast feeding for six months best for babies everywhere.* https://www.who.int/mediacentre/news/statements/2011/breastfeeding_20110115/en/

9. Fangupo, L. J., Heath, A. M., Williams, S. M., et al. (2016, October). A baby-led approach to eating solids and risk of choking. *Pediatrics, 138*(4), Article e20160772. doi:10.1542/peds.2016-0772.

10. Williams Erickson, L., Taylor, R. W., Haszard, J. J., et al. (2018). Impact of a modified version of baby-led weaning on infant food and nutrient intakes: The BLISS randomized controlled trial. *Nutrients, 10*(6), 740. doi:10.3390/nu10060740.

11. Tournier, C., Bernad, C., Madrelle, J., et al. (2021). Fostering infant food texture acceptance: A pilot intervention promoting food texture introduction between 8 and 15 months. *Appetite, 158,* 104989. doi:10.1016/j.appet.2020.104989.

12. Coulthard, H., Harris, G., & Emmett, P. (2009). Delayed introduction of lumpy foods to children during the complementary feeding period affects child's food acceptance and feeding at 7 years of age. *Maternal & Child Nutrition, 5*(1), 75–85. doi:10.1111/j.1740-8709.2008.00153.x.

13. Harris, G., & Mason, S. (2017). Are there sensitive periods for food acceptance in infancy? *Current Nutrition Reports, 6*(2), 190–196. doi:10.1007/s13668-017-0203-0.

14. Roberts, G., Bahnson, H. T., Du Toit, G., et al. (2023). Defining the window of opportunity and target populations to prevent peanut allergy. *Journal of Allergy & Clinical Immunology, 151*(5), 1329–1336. doi:10.1016/j.jaci.2022.09.042.

15. Fleischer, D. M., Chan, E. S., Venter, C., et al. (2021). A consensus approach to the primary prevention of food allergy through nutrition: Guidance from the American Academy of Allergy, Asthma, and Immunology; American College of Allergy, Asthma, and Immunology; and the Canadian Society for Allergy and Clinical Immunology. *Journal of Allergy & Clinical Immunology: In Practice, 9*(1), 22–43.e4. doi:10.1016/j.jaip.2020.11.002.

16. Harris, G., & Mason, S. (2017).

17. Bentley, A. (2014).

18. *Time.* (1940, March 18). *Foods: Tin can mother.* https://content.time.com/time/subscriber/article/0,33009,763689,00.html

19. Rapley, G. (2016). Are puréed foods justified for infants of 6 months? What does the evidence tell us? *Journal of Health Visiting, 4*(6), 289–295.

20. World Health Organization. (2023). WHO Guideline for complementary feeding of infants and young children 6–23 months of age. https://www.ncbi.nlm.nih.gov/books/NBK596427/

Chapter Three

1. Harris, G., & Mason, S. (2017). Are there sensitive periods for food acceptance in infancy? *Current Nutrition Reports, 6*(2), 190–196. doi:10.1007/s13668-017-0203-0.

2. Northstone, K., Emmett, P., Nethersole, F., & ALSPAC Study Team (Avon Longitudinal Study of Pregnancy and Childhood). (2001). The effect of age of introduction to lumpy solids on foods eaten and reported feeding difficulties at 6 and 15 months. *Journal of Human Nutrition & Dietetics, 14*(1), 43–54. doi:10.1046/j.1365-277x.2001.00264.x.

3. Coulthard, H., Harris, G., & Emmett, P. (2009). Delayed introduction of lumpy foods to children during the complementary feeding period affects child's food acceptance and feeding at 7 years of age. *Maternal & Child Nutrition, 5*(1), 75–85. doi:10.1111/j.1740-8709.2008.00153.x.

4. Du Toit, G., Roberts, G., Sayre, P. H., et al., & LEAP Study Team (2015). Randomized trial of peanut consumption in infants at risk for peanut allergy. *New England Journal of Medicine, 372*(9), 803–813. doi:10.1056/NEJMoa1414850.

5. Du Toit, G., Sayre, P. H., Roberts, G., et al., & Immune Tolerance Network LEAP-On Study Team. (2016). Effect of avoidance on peanut allergy after early peanut consumption. *New England Journal of Medicine, 374*(15), 1435–1443. doi.org/10.1056/NEJMoa1514209.

6. Keet, C., Pistiner, M., Plesa, M., et al. (2021). Age and eczema severity, but not family history, are major risk factors for peanut allergy in infancy. *Journal of Allergy & Clinical Immunology, 147*(3), 984–991.e5. doi:10.1016/j.jaci.2020.11.033.

7. Roberts, G., Bahnson, H. T., Du Toit, G., et al. (2023). Defining the window of opportunity and target populations to prevent peanut allergy. *Journal of Allergy & Clinical Immunology, 151*(5), 1329–1336. doi:10.1016/j.jaci.2022.09.042.

8. da Costa, S. P., Remijn, L., Weenen, H., et al. (2017). Exposure to texture of foods for 8-month-old infants: Does the size of the pieces matter? *Journal of Texture Studies, 48*(6), 534–540. doi:10.1111/jtxs.12271.

9. Coulthard, H., Harris, G., & Emmett, P. (2010). Long-term consequences of early fruit and vegetable feeding practices in the United Kingdom. *Public Health Nutrition, 13*(12), 2044–2051. doi:10.1017/S1368980010000790.

10. Northstone, K., Emmett, P., Nethersole, F., & ALSPAC Study Team (Avon Longitudinal Study of Pregnancy and Childhood). (2001). The effect of age of introduction to lumpy solids on foods eaten and reported feeding difficulties at 6 and 15 months. *Journal of Human Nutrition & Dietetics, 14*(1), 43–54. doi:10.1046/j.1365-277x.2001.00264.x.

11. Harris, G., & Mason, S. (2017).

12. Du Plessis, L., Kruger, H., & Sweet, L. (2013). II. Complementary feeding: A critical window of opportunity from six months onwards. *South African Journal of Clinical Nutrition, 26*(S), S129–S140.

13. Tournier, C., Bernad, C., Madrelle, J., et al. (2021). Fostering infant food texture acceptance: A pilot intervention promoting food texture introduction between 8 and 15 months. *Appetite, 158,* 104989. doi:10.1016/j.appet.2020.104989.

14. da Costa, S. P., Remijn, L., Weenen, H., et al. (2017).
15. Le Révérend, B. J., Edelson, L. R., & Loret, C. (2014). Anatomical, functional, physiological and behavioural aspects of the development of mastication in early childhood. *British Journal of Nutrition, 111*(3), 403–414. doi:10.1017/S0007114513002699.
16. Arvedson, J. C., Brodsky, L., & Lefton-Greif, M. (2019). *Pediatric swallowing and feeding: Assessment and management* (3rd ed). Plural.
17. Redstone, F., & West, J. F. (2004). The importance of postural control for feeding. *Pediatric Nursing, 30*(2), 97–100.
18. Wilson, E. M., Green, J. R., & Weismer, G. (2012). A kinematic description of the temporal characteristics of jaw motion for early chewing: Preliminary findings. *Journal of Speech, Language, & Hearing Research, 55*(2), 626–638. doi:10.1044/1092-4388(2011/10-0236.
19. Carruth, B. R., & Skinner, J. D. (2002). Feeding behaviors and other motor development in healthy children (2–24 months). *Journal of the American College of Nutrition, 21*(2), 88–96. doi:10.1080/07315724.2002.10719199.
20. Wilson, E. M., & Green, J. R. (2009). The development of jaw motion for mastication. *Early Human Development, 85*(5), 303–311. doi:10.1016/j.earlhumdev.2008.12.003.
21. Arvedson J. C., Brodsky L., & Lefton-Greif M. (2019). *Pediatric swallowing and feeding: Assessment and management.* 3rd ed. New York: Plural Publishing.
22. Harris, G., & Mason, S. (2017).
23. Almaatani, D., Zurbau, A., Khoshnevisan, F., et al. (2023). The association between parents' stress and parental feeding practices and feeding styles: Systematic review and meta-analysis of observational studies. *Maternal & Child Nutrition, 19*(1), Article e13448. doi:10.1111/mcn.13448.
24. Harvey, L., Bryant-Waugh, R., Watkins, B., et al. (2015). Parental perceptions of childhood feeding problems. *Journal of Child Health Care: For Professionals Working with Children in the Hospital & Community, 19*(3), 392–401. doi:10.1177/1367493513509422.

Chapter Four

1. Karen, R. (1998). *Becoming attached: First relationships and how they shape our capacity to love.* Oxford University Press.
2. Adolph, K. E. (2008). Learning to move. *Current Directions in Psychological Science, 17*(3), 213–218. doi:10.1111/j.1467-8721.2008.00577.x.
3. Adolph, K. E. (2008).
4. Tylka, T. L., Lumeng, J. C., & Eneli, I. U. (2015). Maternal intuitive eating as a moderator of the association between concern about child weight and restrictive child feeding. *Appetite, 95,* 158–165. doi:10.1016/j.appet.2015.06.023.
5. Savage, J. S., Fisher, J. O., & Birch, L. L. (2007). Parental influence on eating behavior: Conception to adolescence. *Journal of Law, Medicine & Ethics, 35*(1), 22–34. doi:10.1111/j.1748-720X.2007.00111.x.
6. Fildes, A., van Jaarsveld, C. H., Llewellyn, C., et al. (2015). Parental control over feeding in infancy. Influence of infant weight, appetite and feeding method. *Appetite, 91,* 101–106. doi:10.1016/j.appet.2015.04.004.

7. Øverby, N. C., Hillesund, E. R., Røed, M., et al. (2020). Association between parental feeding practices and shared family meals. The Food4toddlers study. *Food & Nutrition Research, 64*. doi:10.29219/fnr.v64.4456.

8. León, M. P., González-Martí, I., & Contreras-Jordán, O. R. (2021). What do children think of their perceived and ideal bodies? Understandings of body image at early ages: A mixed study. *International Journal of Environmental Research & Public Health, 18*(9), 4871. doi:10.3390/ijerph18094871.

9. Eli, K., Howell, K., Fisher, P. A., et al. (2014). "Those comments last forever": Parents and grandparents of preschoolers recount how they became aware of their own body weights as children. *PLoS One, 9*(11), Article e111974. doi:10.1371/journal.pone.0111974.

10. Nehls, S., Losse, E., Enzensberger, C., et al. (2024). Time-sensitive changes in the maternal brain and their influence on mother-child attachment. *Translational Psychiatry, 14*, 84. doi:10.1038/s41398-024-02805-2.

11. Robson, S. M., McCullough, M. B., Rex, S., et al. (2020). Family meal frequency, diet, and family functioning: A systematic review with meta-analyses. *Journal of Nutrition Education & Behavior, 52*(5), 553–564. doi:10.1016/j.jneb.2019.12.012.

12. Harbec, M., & Pagani, L. S. (2018). Associations between early family meal environment quality and later well-being in school-age children. *Journal of Developmental & Behavioral Pediatrics, 39*(2), 136–143. doi:10.1097/DBP.0000000000000520.

13. Cook, R., Bird, G., Catmur, C., et al. (2014). Mirror neurons: From origin to function. *Behavioral & Brain Sciences, 37*(2), 177–192. doi:10.1017/S0140525X13000903.

14. Marshall, P. J., & Meltzoff, A. N. (2014). Neural mirroring mechanisms and imitation in human infants. *Philosophical Transactions of the Royal Society B: Biological Sciences, 369*(1644), 20130620. doi:10.1098/rstb.2013.0620.

15. Harbec, M., & Pagani, L. S. (2018).

Chapter Five

1. Karen, R. (1998). *Becoming attached: First relationships and how they shape our capacity to love*. Oxford University Press.

2. Moriceau, S., & Sullivan, R. M. (2005). Neurobiology of infant attachment. *Developmental Psychobiology: Journal of the International Society for Developmental Psychobiology, 47*(3), 230–242. doi:10.1002/dev.20093.

3. Black, M. M., & Aboud, F. E. (2011). Responsive feeding is embedded in a theoretical framework of responsive parenting. *Journal of Nutrition, 141*(3), 490–494. doi:10.3945/jn.110.129973.

4. Stern, J. A., Barbarin, O., & Cassidy, J. (2022). Working toward anti-racist perspectives in attachment theory, research, and practice. *Attachment & Human Development, 24*(3), 392–422. doi:10.1080/14616734.2021.1976933.

5. Causadias, J. M., Morris, K. S., Cárcamo, R. A., et al. (2022). Attachment research and anti-racism: learning from Black and Brown scholars. *Attachment & Human Development, 24*(3), 366–372. doi:10.1080/14616734.2021.1976936.

6. Satter, E. (2012). *Child of mine: Feeding with love and good sense*. Bull.

7. Mermelshtine, R. (2017). Parent-child learning interactions: A review of the

literature on scaffolding. *British Journal of Educational Psychology, 87*(2), 241–254. doi:10.1111/bjep.12147.

8. Gillespie, L. G., & Greenberg, J. D. (2017). Empowering infants' and toddlers' learning through scaffolding. *YC Young Children, 72*(2), 90–93.

9. Burke, J. P. (1977). A clinical perspective on motivation: Pawn versus origin. *American Journal of Occupational Therapy, 31,* 254–258.

10. Mermelshtine, R. (2017).

Chapter Six

1. Centers for Disease Control and Prevention, National Center for Health Statistics. National Vital Statistics System, Mortality 1999–2020 on CDC WONDER Online Database, released in 2021. Data are from the Multiple Cause of Death Files, 1999–2020, as compiled from data provided by the fifty-seven vital statistics jurisdictions through the Vital Statistics Cooperative Program. Retrieved January 3, 2024, from http://wonder.cdc.gov/ucd-icd10.html

2. Northstone, K., Emmett, P., Nethersole, F., & ALSPAC Study Team (Avon Longitudinal Study of Pregnancy and Childhood). (2001). The effect of age of introduction to lumpy solids on foods eaten and reported feeding difficulties at 6 and 15 months. *Journal of Human Nutrition & Dietetics, 14*(1), 43–54. doi:10.1046/j.1365-277x.2001.00264.x.

3. Coulthard, H., Harris, G., & Emmett, P. (2009). Delayed introduction of lumpy foods to children during the complementary feeding period affects child's food acceptance and feeding at 7 years of age. *Maternal & Child Nutrition, 5*(1), 75–85. doi:10.1111/j.1740-8709.2008.00153.x.

4. Le Révérend, B. J., Edelson, L. R., & Loret, C. (2014). Anatomical, functional, physiological and behavioural aspects of the development of mastication in early childhood. *British Journal of Nutrition, 111*(3), 403–414. doi:10.1017/S0007114513002699.

5. Tournier, C., Demonteil, L., Ksiazek, E., et al. (2021). Factors associated with food texture acceptance in 4- to 36-month-old French children: Findings from a survey study. *Frontiers in Nutrition, 7,* 616484. doi:10.3389/fnut.2020.616484.

6. Larrick, B. M., Dwyer, J. T., Erdman, J. W., et al. (2022). An updated framework for industry funding of food and nutrition research: Managing financial conflicts and scientific integrity. *Journal of Nutrition, 152*(8), 1812–1818. doi:10.1093/jn/nxac106.

7. Centers for Disease Control and Prevention, National Center for Health Statistics.

8. Centers for Disease Control and Prevention, National Center for Health Statistics.

9. Wake, M., Hesketh, K., & Lucas, J. (2000). Teething and tooth eruption in infants: A cohort study. *Pediatrics, 106*(6), 1374–1379. doi:10.1542/peds.106.6.1374.

10. Fangupo, L. J., Heath, A. M., Williams, S. M., et al. (2016). A baby-led approach to eating solids and risk of choking. *Pediatrics, 138*(4), Article e20160772. doi:10.1542/peds.2016-0772.

11. Sakamoto, M., Watanabe, Y., Edahiro, A., et al. (2018). Self-feeding ability as a predictor of mortality Japanese nursing home residents: A two-year

longitudinal study. *Journal of Nutrition, Health & Aging, 23*(2), 157–164. doi:10
.1007/s12603-018-1125-2.

12. Smith, C. H., Teo, Y., & Simpson, S. (2013). An observational study of adults
with Down syndrome eating independently. *Dysphagia, 29*(1), 52–60. doi:10
.1007/s00455-013-9479-4.

13. Shune, S. E., Moon, J. B., & Goodman, S. S. (2016). The effects of age and
preoral sensorimotor cues on anticipatory mouth movement during
swallowing. *Journal of Speech, Language, & Hearing Research, 59*(2), 195–205. doi:10
.1044/2015_JSLHR-S-15-0138.

14. Corbin-Lewis, K., Liss, J. M., & Sciortino, K. (2005). *Clinical anatomy and physiology
of the swallowing mechanism.* Clifton Park, NY: Thompson.

15. Sakamoto, M., Watanabe, Y., Edahiro, A., et al. (2018).

16. Smith, C. H., Teo, Y., & Simpson, S. (2013).

17. Shune, S. E., Moon, J. B., & Goodman, S. S. (2016).

18. Arvedson, J. C., Brodsky, L., & Lefton-Greif, M. (2019). *Pediatric swallowing and
feeding: Assessment and management* (3rd ed). Plural.

19. Fangupo, L. J., Heath, A. M., Williams, S. M., et al. (2016).

20. Corbin-Lewis, K., Liss, J. M., & Sciortino, K. (2005).

21. Corbin-Lewis, K., Liss, J. M., & Sciortino, K. (2005).

22. Lorenzoni, G., Hochdorn, A., Beltrame Vriz, G., et al. (2022). Regulatory and
educational initiatives to prevent food choking injuries in children: An
overview of the current approaches. *Frontiers in Public Health, 10,* 830876.
doi:10.3389/fpubh.2022.830876.

23. Le Révérend, B. J., Edelson, L. R., & Loret, C. (2014).

24. Ertekin, Ç., Keskin, A., Kıylıoğlu, N., et al. (2001). The effect of head and neck
positions on oropharyngeal swallowing: A clinical and electrophysiologic
study. *Archives of Physical Medicine & Rehabilitation, 82*(9), 1255–1260. doi:10.1053/
apmr.2001.25156.

25. Centers for Disease Control and Prevention, National Center for Health Statistics.

26. Consumer Product Safety Commission. (2024, April). National Electronic
Injury Surveillance System 2004–2023. NEISS Online Database. Retrieved
August 13, 2024, from https://www.cpsc.gov/cgibin/NEISSQuery/home.aspx

27. Harris, C. S., Baker, S. P., Smith, G. A., et al. (1984). Childhood asphyxiation by
food: A national analysis and overview. *Journal of the American Medical
Association, 251*(17), 2231–2235.

28. Committee on Injury, Violence, and Poison Prevention. (2010). Prevention of
choking among children. *Pediatrics, 125*(3), 601–607. doi:10.1542/
peds.2009-2862.

29. Correia, L., Sousa, A. R., Capitão, C., & Pedro, A. R. (2024). Complementary
feeding approaches and risk of choking: A systematic review. *Journal of Pediatric
Gastroenterology and Nutrition, 79*(5), 934–942. doi.org/10.1002/jpn3.12298.

Chapter Seven

1. World Health Organization. (2011). *Exclusive breast feeding for six months best for
babies everywhere.* https://www.who.int/mediacentre/news/statements/2011/
breastfeeding_20110115/en/

2. Meek, J. Y., & Noble, L. (2022). Section on breastfeeding; Policy statement: Breastfeeding and the use of human milk. *Pediatrics, 150*(1), Article e2022057988. doi:10.1542/peds.2022-057988.

3. Wright, C. M., Cameron, K., Tsiaka, M., et al. (2011). Is baby-led weaning feasible? When do babies first reach out for and eat finger foods? *Maternal & Child Nutrition, 7*(1), 27–33. doi:10.1111/j.1740-8709.2010.00274.x.

4. Cleary, J., Dalton, S., Harman, A., et al. (2020). Current practice in the introduction of solid foods for preterm infants. *Public Health Nutrition, 23*(1), 94–101. doi:10.1017/S1368980019002337.

5. Palmer, D. J., & Makrides, M. (2012). Introducing solid foods to preterm infants in developed countries. *Annals of Nutrition & Metabolism, 60*(Suppl 2), 31–38. doi:10.1159/000335336.

6. Brown, A., & Harries, V. (2015). Infant sleep and night feeding patterns during later infancy: Association with breastfeeding frequency, daytime complementary food intake, and infant weight. *Breastfeeding Medicine, 10*(5), 246–252. doi:10.1089/bfm.2014.0153.

7. Nelson, S. P., Chen, E. H., Syniar, G. M., et al. (1997). Prevalence of symptoms of gastroesophageal reflux during infancy. A pediatric practice-based survey. Pediatric Practice Research Group. *Archives of Pediatrics & Adolescent Medicine, 151*(6), 569–572. doi:10.1001/archpedi.1997.02170430035007.

8. Hegar, B., Satari, D. H., Sjarif, D. R., et al. (2013). Regurgitation and gastroesophageal reflux disease in six to nine months old Indonesian infants. *Pediatric Gastroenterology, Hepatology & Nutrition, 16*(4), 240–247. doi:10.5223/pghn.2013.16.4.240.

9. Campanozzi, A., Boccia, G., Pensabene, L., et al. (2009). Prevalence and natural history of gastroesophageal reflux: pediatric prospective survey. *Pediatrics, 123*(3), 779–783. doi:10.1542/peds.2007-3569.

10. Coulthard, H., Harris, G., & Fogel, A. (2014). Exposure to vegetable variety in infants weaned at different ages. *Appetite, 78*, 89–94. doi:10.1016/j.appet.2014.03.021.

11. Fangupo, L. J., Heath, A. M., Williams, S. M., et al. (2016, October). A baby-led approach to eating solids and risk of choking. *Pediatrics, 138*(4), Article e20160772. doi:10.1542/peds.2016-0772.

12. Ertekin, C., Keskin, A., Kiylioglu, N., et al. (2001). The effect of head and neck positions on oropharyngeal swallowing: A clinical and electrophysiologic study. *Archives of Physical Medicine & Rehabilitation, 82*(9), 1255–1260. doi:10.1053/apmr.2001.25156.

13. Shune, S. E., Moon, J. B., & Goodman, S. S. (2016). The effects of age and preoral sensorimotor cues on anticipatory mouth movement during swallowing. *Journal of Speech, Language, & Hearing Research, 59*(2), 195–205. doi:10.1044/2015_JSLHR-S-15-0138.

14. Sasegbon, A., & Hamdy, S. (2017). The anatomy and physiology of normal and abnormal swallowing in oropharyngeal dysphagia. *Neurogastroenterology & Motility, 29*(11). doi:10.1111/nmo.13100.

15. World Health Organization. (2023). WHO Guideline for complementary

feeding of infants and young children 6–23 months of age. https://www.ncbi
.nlm.nih.gov/books/NBK596427/
16. Meek, J. Y., & Noble, L. (2022).

Chapter Eight

1. Sakaguchi, K., Mehta, N. R., Maruyama, T., et al. (2023). Effect of sitting posture
   with and without sole-ground contact on chewing stability and masticatory
   performance. *Journal of Oral Science, 65*(4), 251–256. doi:10.2334/josnusd.23-0172.
2. Moriceau, S., & Sullivan, R. M. (2005). Neurobiology of infant attachment.
   *Developmental Psychobiology: The Journal of the International Society for Developmental
   Psychobiology, 47*(3), 230–242. doi:10.1002/dev.20093.
3. Karen, R. (1998). *Becoming attached: First relationships and how they shape our capacity
   to love.* Oxford University Press.
4. Sakaguchi, K., Mehta, N. R., Maruyama, T., et al. (2023).
5. Uesugi, Y., Ihara, Y., Yuasa, K., et al. (2019). Sole-ground contact and sitting leg
   position influence suprahyoid and sternocleidomastoid muscle activity during
   swallowing of liquids. *Clinical & Experimental Dental Research, 5*(5), 505–512.
   doi:10.1002/cre2.216.
6. Morris, S. E., & Klein, M. D. (2000). *Pre-feeding skills* (2nd ed). Therapy Skill
   Builders.
7. National Electronic Injury Surveillance System (NEISS). (2021). U.S. Consumer
   Product Safety Commission.
8. Consumer Product Safety Commission. (2024, April). National Electronic
   Injury Surveillance System 2004–2023. NEISS Online Database. Retrieved
   August 13, 2024, from https://www.cpsc.gov/cgibin/NEISSQuery/home.aspx
9. Black, M. M., & Aboud, F. E. (2011). Responsive feeding is embedded in a
   theoretical framework of responsive parenting. *Journal of Nutrition, 141*(3),
   490–494. doi:10.3945/jn.110.129973.

Chapter Nine

1. FoodSafety.gov. (2013, September 21). *People at risk: Children under five.* https://
   www.foodsafety.gov/people-at-risk/children-under-five
2. Centers for Disease Control and Prevention. (2024, April 29). *About four steps to
   food safety.* https://cdc.gov/food-safety/prevention/
3. Health Canada. (2015, March). *Safe food handling for children ages 5 and under.*
   Retrieved November 5, 2021. from https://www.canada.ca/content/dam/hc-sc/
   documents/services/food-safety-vulnerable-populations/food-safety
   -vulnerable-populations/children-under-5-moins-enfant-eng.pdf
4. Food Standards Agency. (2024, May). *Salmonella.* Retrieved August 5, 2024,
   from https://www.food.gov.uk/safety-hygiene/salmonella
5. California Office of Environmental Health Hazard Assessment. (2019, May 24).
   Mercury in fish and shellfish. https://oehha.ca.gov/fish/mercury-fish-information
   -people-who-eat-fish
6. Augustin, J., Augustin, E., Cutrufelli, R. L., et al. (1992). Alcohol retention in
   food preparation. *Journal of the American Dietetic Association, 92*(4), 486–488.

7. Gaw, C. E., & Osterhoudt, K. C. (2020, December 10). Babies can get sick from alcohol. https://injury.research.chop.edu/blog/posts/babies-can-get-sick -alcohol

8. Gaw, C. E., Lim, C. G., Korenoski, A. S., et al. (2021). Beverage ethanol exposures among infants reported to United States poison control centers. *Clinical Toxicology, 59*(7), 619–627. doi:10.1080/15563650.2020.1843660.

9. Gupta, P. M., Hamner, H. C., Suchdev, P. S., et al. (2017). Iron status of toddlers, nonpregnant females, and pregnant females in the United States. *American Journal of Clinical Nutrition, 106*(Suppl 6), 1640S—1646S. doi:10.3945/ajcn.117 .155978.

10. Moscheo, C., Licciardello, M., Samperi, P., et al. (2022). New insights into iron deficiency anemia in children: A practical review. *Metabolites, 12*(4), 289. doi:10.3390/metabo12040289.

11. van der Merwe, L. F., & Eussen, S. R. (2017). Iron status of young children in Europe. *American Journal of Clinical Nutrition, 106*(Suppl 6), 1663S–1671S. doi:10.3945/ajcn.117.156018.

12. Bates, M., Gupta, P. M., Cogswell, M. E., et al. (2020). Iron content of commercially available infant and toddler foods in the United States, 2015. *Nutrients, 12*(8), 2439. doi:10.3390/nu12082439.

13. Katiforis, I., Fleming, E. A., Haszard, J. J., et al. (2021). Energy, sugars, iron, and vitamin B12 content of commercial infant food pouches and other commercial infant foods on the New Zealand market. *Nutrients, 13*(2), 657. doi:10.3390/ nu13020657.

Chapter Ten

1. Fangupo, L. J., Heath, A. M., Williams, S. M., et al. (2016, October). A baby-led approach to eating solids and risk of choking. *Pediatrics, 138*(4), Article e20160772. doi:10.1542/peds.2016-0772.

2. Shune, S. E., Moon, J. B., & Goodman, S. S. (2016). The effects of age and preoral sensorimotor cues on anticipatory mouth movement during swallowing. *Journal of Speech, Language, & Hearing Research, 59*(2), 195–205. doi:10.1044/2015_jslhr-s-15-0138.

3. Sakamoto, M., Watanabe, Y., Edahiro, A., et al. (2018). Self-feeding ability as a predictor of mortality Japanese nursing home residents: A two-year longitudinal study. *Journal of Nutrition, Health & Aging, 23*(2), 157–164. doi:10.1007/s12603-018-1125-2.

4. Simione, M., Loret, C., Le Révérend, B., et al. (2018). Differing structural properties of foods affect the development of mandibular control and muscle coordination in infants and young children. *Physiology & Behavior, 186*, 62–72. doi:10.1016/j.physbeh.2018.01.009.

5. Smith, C. H., Teo, Y., & Simpson, S. (2013). An observational study of adults with Down syndrome eating independently. *Dysphagia, 29*(1), 52–60. doi:10.1007/s00455-013-9479-4.

6. World Health Organization. (2023). WHO Guideline for complementary feeding of infants and young children 6–23 months of age. https://www.ncbi .nlm.nih.gov/books/NBK596427/

7. Hill, L. F., Lowe, C. U., Smith, C. A., et al. (1958). On the feeding of solid foods to infants. *Pediatrics, 21,* 685–692.

8. Samady, W., Campbell, E., Aktas, O. N., et al. (2020). Recommendations on complementary food introduction among pediatric practitioners. *JAMA Network Open, 3*(8), Article e2013070. doi:10.1001/jamanetworkopen.2020.13070.

9. Trulsson, M., & Johansson, R. S. (2002). Orofacial mechanoreceptors in humans: Encoding characteristics and responses during natural orofacial behaviors. *Behavioural Brain Research, 135*(1–2), 27–33. doi:10.1016/s0166-4328(02)00151-1.

10. Simione, M., Loret, C., Le Révérend, B., et al. (2018).

11. Takahashi, T., Miyamoto, T., Terao, A., et al. (2007). Cerebral activation related to the control of mastication during changes in food hardness. *Neuroscience, 145,* 791–794. doi:10.1016/j.neuroscience.2006.12.044.

12. Jadcherla, S. R., Hogan, W. J., & Shaker, R. (2010). Physiology and pathophysiology of glottic reflexes and pulmonary aspiration: From neonates to adults. *Seminars in Respiratory & Critical Care Medicine, 31*(5), 554–560. doi:10.1055/s-0030-1265896.

13. Bayley, N. (2006). Bayley scales of infant and toddler development. Psychological Corporation. [Bayley Scales of Infant and Toddler Development is a formal assessment tool for diagnosing developmental delays in childhood.]

14. Fangupo, L. J., Heath, A. M., Williams, S. M., et al. (2016).

15. Geisel, E. G. (1991). Effect of food texture on the development of chewing of children between six months and two years of age. *Developmental Medicine & Child Neurology, 3,* 69–79. doi:10.1111/j.1469-8749.1991.tb14786.x.

16. da Costa, S. P., Remijn, L., Weenen, H., et al. (2017). Exposure to texture of foods for 8-month-old infants: Does the size of the pieces matter? *Journal of Texture Studies, 48*(6), 534–540. doi:10.1111/jtxs.12271.

17. Harris, G., & Mason, S. (2017). Are there sensitive periods for food acceptance in infancy? *Current Nutrition Reports, 6*(2), 190–196. doi:10.1007/s13668-017-0203-0.

18. Northstone, K., Emmett, P., Nethersole, F., & ALSPAC Study Team (Avon Longitudinal Study of Pregnancy and Childhood). (2001). The effect of age of introduction to lumpy solids on foods eaten and reported feeding difficulties at 6 and 15 months. *Journal of Human Nutrition & Dietetics, 14*(1), 43–54. doi:10.1046/j.1365-277x.2001.00264.x.

19. Coulthard, H., Harris, G., & Emmett, P. (2009). Delayed introduction of lumpy foods to children during the complementary feeding period affects child's food acceptance and feeding at 7 years of age. *Maternal & Child Nutrition, 5*(1), 75–85. doi:10.1111/j.1740-8709.2008.00153.x.

Chapter Eleven

1. Scaglioni, S., De Cosmi, V., Ciappolino, V., et al. (2018). Factors influencing children's eating behaviours. *Nutrients, 10*(6), 706. doi:10.3390/nu10060706.

2. Tylka, T. L., Lumeng, J. C., & Eneli, I. U. (2015). Maternal intuitive eating as a moderator of the association between concern about child weight and restrictive child feeding. *Appetite, 95,* 158–165. doi:10.1016/j.appet.2015.06.023.

3. Visser, M. (2015). *The rituals of dinner: The origins, evolution, eccentricities, and meaning of table manners.* Open Road Media.

4. Thompson, S. D., & Raisor, J. M. (2013). Individualizing in early childhood: The what, why, and how of differentiated approaches: Meeting the sensory needs of young children. *YC Young Children, 68*(2), 34–43. https://issuu.com/naeyc/docs/meeting_sensory_needs_thompson_0513

5. Nekitsing, C., Hetherington, M. M., & Blundell-Birtill, P. (2018). Developing healthy food preferences in preschool children through taste exposure, sensory learning, and nutrition education. *Current Obesity Reports, 7,* 60–67. doi:10.1007/s13679-018-0297-8.

6. Cappellotto, M., & Olsen, A. (2021). Food texture acceptance, sensory sensitivity, and food neophobia in children and their parents. *Foods, 10*(10), 2327. doi:10.3390/foods10102327.

7. Nederkoorn, C., Houben, K., & Havermans, R. C. (2019). Taste the texture. The relation between subjective tactile sensitivity, mouthfeel and picky eating in young adults. *Appetite, 136,* 58–161. doi:10.1016/j.appet.2019.01.015.

8. Nederkoorn, C., Jansen, A., & Havermans, R. C. (2015). Feel your food. The influence of tactile sensitivity on picky eating in children. *Appetite, 84,* 7–10. doi:10.1016/j.appet.2014.09.014.

Chapter Fourteen

1. Food and Agriculture Organization of the United Nations and World Health Organization. (2022). Risk assessment of food allergens. Part 1—Review and validation of Codex Alimentarius priority allergen list through risk assessment. Meeting report. Food Safety and Quality Series No. 14.

2. Vickery, B. P., Berglund, J. P., Burk, C. M., et al. (2017). Early oral immunotherapy in peanut-allergic preschool children is safe and highly effective. *Journal of Allergy & Clinical Immunology, 139*(1), 173–181.e8. doi:10.1016/j.jaci.2016.05.027.

3. Gupta, R.S., Warren, C.M., Smith, B.M., Blumenstock, J.A., Jiang, J., et al. (2018). The public health impact of parent-reported childhood food allergies in the United States. *Pediatrics, 142*(6):e20181235.

4. Food Allergy Research & Education (FARE). *Facts & Statistics.* Retrieved April 17, 2024, from https://www.foodallergy.org/resources/facts-and-statistics

5. Du Toit, G., Katz, Y., Sasieni, P., et al. (2008). Early consumption of peanuts in infancy is associated with a low prevalence of peanut allergy. *Journal of Allergy & Clinical Immunology, 122*(5), 984–991. doi:10.1016/j.jaci.2008.08.039.

6. Du Toit, G., Roberts, G., Sayre, P. H., Bahnson, H.T., Radulovic, S., Santos, A.F., et al. (2015). LEAP Study Team. Randomized trial of peanut consumption in infants at risk for peanut allergy. *New England Journal of Medicine, 372*(9):803–13. Erratum in: *New England Journal of Medicine,* 2016 Jul 28;375(4):398. doi:10.1056/NEJMx150044.

7. Food Allergy Research & Education (FARE). (n.d.). *Learning early about peanut allergy (LEAP).* Retrieved April 17, 2024, from https://www.foodallergy.org/resources/learning-early-about-peanut-allergy-leap

8. Perkin, M. R., Logan, K., Marrs, T., et al., & EAT Study Team (2016). Enquiring About Tolerance (EAT) study: Feasibility of an early allergenic food introduction regimen. *Journal of Allergy and Clinical Immunology, 137*(5), 1477–1486. doi.org/10.1016/j.jaci.2015.12.1322.

9. Natsume, O., Kabashima, S., Nakazato, J., et al. (2017). Two-step egg introduction for prevention of egg allergy in high-risk infants with eczema (PETIT): A randomised, double-blind, placebo-controlled trial. *Lancet, 389*(10066), 276–286. doi:10.1016/S0140-6736(16)31418-0.

10. Togias, A., Cooper, S. F., Acebal, M. L., et al. (2017). Addendum guidelines for the prevention of peanut allergy in the United States: Report of the National Institute of Allergy and Infectious Diseases-sponsored expert panel. *Journal of Allergy & Clinical Immunology, 139*, 29–44. doi:10.1016/j.jaci.2016 .10.010.

11. Fleischer, D. M., Chan, E. S., Venter, C., et al. (2021). A consensus approach to the primary prevention of food allergy through nutrition: guidance from the American Academy of Allergy, Asthma, and Immunology; American College of Allergy, Asthma, and Immunology; and the Canadian Society for Allergy and Clinical Immunology. *Journal of Allergy & Clinical Immunology: In Practice, 9*(1), 22–43.e4. doi:10.1016/j.jaip.2020.11.002.

12. Joshi, P. A., Smith, J., Vale, S., & Campbell, D. E. (2019). The Australasian Society of Clinical Immunology and Allergy infant feeding for allergy prevention guidelines. *Medical Journal of Australia, 210*(2), 89–93. doi.org/10 .5694/mja2.12102.

13. Tham, E. H., Shek, L. P., Van Bever, H. P., & Asia Pacific Academy of Pediatric Allergy, Respirology & Immunology (APAPARI). (2018). Early introduction of allergenic foods for the prevention of food allergy from an Asian perspective—An Asia Pacific Association of Pediatric Allergy, Respirology & Immunology (APAPARI) consensus statement. *Pediatric Allergy & Immunology, 29*, 18–27. doi:10.1111/pai.12820.

14. Abrams, E. M., Hildebrand, K., Blair, B., et al. (2019). Timing of introduction of allergenic solids for infants at high risk. *Paediatrics & Child Health, 24*, 56–57. doi:10.1093/pch/pxy195.

15. Ebisawa, M., Ito, K., Fujisawa, T., Committee for Japanese Pediatric Guideline for Food Allergy, Japanese Society of Pediatric Allergy and Clinical Immunology, & Japanese Society of Allergology. (2020). Japanese guidelines for food allergy 2020. *Allergology, 69*, 370–386. doi:10.1016/j.alit.2020.03.004.

16. Halken, S., Muraro, A., de Silva, D., et al., & European Academy of Allergy and Clinical Immunology Food Allergy and Anaphylaxis Guidelines Group. (2021). EAACI guideline: Preventing the development of food allergy in infants and young children (2020 update). *Pediatric Allergy & Immunology, 32*, 843–858. doi:10.1111/pai.13496.

17. Soriano, V. X., Peters, R. L., Ponsonby, A. L., et al. (2019). Earlier ingestion of peanut after changes to infant feeding guidelines: The EarlyNuts study. *Journal of Allergy & Clinical Immunology, 144*(5), 1327–1335.e5. doi:10.1016/j.jaci.2019.07 .032.

18. Gupta, R. S., Walkner, M. M., Greenhawt, M., et al. (2016). Food allergy sensitization and presentation in siblings of food allergic children. *Journal of Allergy & Clinical Immunology: In Practice, 4*(5), 956–962. doi:10.1016/j.jaip.2016.04.009.

19. Keet, C., Pistiner, M., Plesa, M., et al. (2021). Age and eczema severity, but not family history, are major risk factors for peanut allergy in infancy. *Journal of Allergy & Clinical Immunology, 147*(3), 984–991.e5. doi:10.1016/j.jaci.2020.11.033.

20. Gupta, R. S., Walkner, M. M., Greenhawt, M., et al. (2016).

21. Fleischer, D. M., Chan, E. S., Venter, C., et al. (2021).

22. Kvenshagen, B., Jacobsen, M., & Halvorsen, R. (2009). Atopic dermatitis in premature and term children. *Archives of Disease in Childhood, 94*(3), 202–205. doi:10.1136/adc.2008.142869.

23. Fleischer, D. M., Chan, E. S., Venter, C., et al. (2021).

24. Roberts, G., Bahnson, H. T., Du Toit, G., et al. (2023).

25. Keet, C., Pistiner, M., Plesa, M., et al. (2021).

26. Food Allergy Research & Education (FARE). (n.d.). *What is a food allergy?* Retrieved April 17, 2024, from https://www.foodallergy.org/resources/what-food-allergy

27. Sicherer, S. H., Wood, R. A., Stablein, D., et al. (2010). Immunologic features of infants with milk or egg allergy enrolled in an observational study (Consortium of Food Allergy Research) of food allergy. *Journal of Allergy & Clinical Immunology, 125*(5), 1077–1083.e8. doi:10.1016/j.jaci.2010.02.038.

28. Nowak-Węgrzyn, A., Chehade, M., Groetch, M. E., et al. (2017). International consensus guidelines for the diagnosis and management of food protein–induced enterocolitis syndrome: Executive summary—Workgroup Report of the Adverse Reactions to Foods Committee, American Academy of Allergy, Asthma & Immunology. *Journal of Allergy & Clinical Immunology, 139*(4), 1111–1126.e4. doi:10.1016/j.jaci.2016.12.966.

29. Storhaug, C. L., Fosse, S. K., & Fadnes, L. T. (2017). Country, regional, and global estimates for lactose malabsorption in adults: a systematic review and meta-analysis. *Lancet. Gastroenterology & Hepatology, 2*(10), 738–746. doi:10.1016/S2468-1253(17)30154-1.

30. Vandenplas, Y., Broekaert, I., Domellöf, M., et al. (2023). An ESPGHAN position paper on the diagnosis, management and prevention of cow's milk allergy. *Journal of Pediatric Gastroenterology & Nutrition.* doi:10.1097/MPG.0000000000003897.

31. Food Allergy Research & Education (FARE). (n.d.) *Recognizing and treating reaction symptoms.* Retrieved April 17, 2024, from https://www.foodallergy.org/resources/recognizing-and-treating-reaction-symptoms

32. Emmert, V., Lendvai-Emmert, D., Eklics, K., Prémusz, V., Tóth, G.P. (2023). Current Practice in Pediatric Cow's Milk Protein Allergy-Immunological Features and Beyond. *International Journal of Molecular Sciences, 6*;24(5):5025. doi:10.3390/ijms24055025.

33. Roberts, G., Bahnson, H. T., Du Toit, G., et al. (2023, May). Defining the window of opportunity and target populations to prevent peanut allergy. *Journal of Allergy & Clinical Immunology, 151*(5), 1329–1336. doi:10.1016/j.jaci.2022.09.042.

Chapter Fifteen

1. Breij, L. M., Mulder, M. T., van Vark-van der Zee, L. C., et al. (2017). Appetite-regulating hormones in early life and relationships with type of feeding and body composition in healthy term infants. *European Journal of Nutrition, 56*(4), 1725–1732. doi:10.1007/s00394-016-1219-8.

2. Zhao, F., Sun, Y., Zhang, Y., et al. (2023). Comparison of mothers' perceptions of hunger cues in 3-month-old infant under different feeding methods. *BMC Public Health, 23*(1), 444. doi:10.1186/s12889-023-15325-3.

3. Hodges, E. A., Wasser, H. M., Colgan, B. K., et al. (2016). Development of feeding cues during infancy and toddlerhood. *MCN: The American Journal of Maternal/Child Nursing, 41,* 244–251. doi:10.1097/NMC.0000000000000251.

4. McNally, J., Hugh-Jones, S., Caton, S., et al. (2016). Communicating hunger and satiation in the first 2 years of life: a systematic review. *Maternal & Child Nutrition, 12*(2), 205–228. doi:10.1111/mcn.12230.

5. Hodges, E. A., Propper, C. B., Estrem, H., et al. (2020). Feeding during infancy: interpersonal behavior, physiology, and obesity risk. *Child Development Perspectives, 14*(3), 185–191. doi:10.1111/cdep.12376.

6. Yeung, A. Y., & Tadi, P. (2022). *Physiology, obesity neurohormonal appetite and satiety control.* StatPearls. https://www.ncbi.nlm.nih.gov/books/NBK555906/

7. Hodges, E. A., Propper, C. B., Estrem, H., et al. (2020).

8. Bouret, S. G. (2009). Early life origins of obesity: Role of hypothalamic programming. *Journal of Pediatric Gastroenterology & Nutrition, 48,* S31–S38. doi:10.1097/MPG.0b013e3181977375.

9. Savino, F., Lupica, M. M., Liguori, S. A., et al. (2012). Ghrelin and feeding behaviour in preterm infants. *Early Human Development, 88*(Suppl 1), S51–S55. doi:10.1016/j.earlhumdev.2011.12.028.

10. Breij, L. M., Mulder, M. T., van Vark-van der Zee, L. C., et al. (2017). Appetite-regulating hormones in early life and relationships with type of feeding and body composition in healthy term infants. *European Journal of Nutrition, 56*(4), 1725–1732. doi:10.1007/s00394-016-1219-8.

11. Gasmi, A., Nasreen, A., Menzel, A., et al. (2022). Neurotransmitters regulation and food intake: The role of dietary sources in neurotransmission. *Molecules, 28*(1), 210. doi:10.3390/molecules28010210.

12. McNally, J., Hugh-Jones, S., & Hetherington, M. M. (2020). "An invisible map"—maternal perceptions of hunger, satiation and 'enough' in the context of baby led and traditional complementary feeding practices. *Appetite, 148,* 104608. doi:10.1016/j.appet.2020.104608.

13. Pérez-Escamilla, R., Jimenez, E. Y., & Dewey, K. G. (2021). Responsive feeding recommendations: Harmonizing integration into dietary guidelines for infants and young children. *Current Developments in Nutrition, 5*(6), nzab076. doi:10.1093/cdn/nzab076.

14. Burnette, C. B., Hazzard, V. M., Hahn, S. L., et al. (2022). Like parent, like child? Intuitive eating among emerging adults and their parents. *Appetite, 176,* 106132. doi:10.1016/j.appet.2022.106132.

15. Rodgers, R. F., Hazzard, V. M., Franko, D. L., et al. (2022). Intuitive eating

among parents: Associations with the home food and meal environment. *Journal of the Academy of Nutrition & Dietetics, 122*(7), 13361344. doi:10.1016/j.jand.2022.01.009.

16. Christoph, M., Järvelä-Reijonen, E., Hooper, L., et al. (2021). Longitudinal associations between intuitive eating and weight-related behaviors in a population-based sample of young adults. *Appetite, 160,* 105093. doi:10.1016/j.appet.2021.105093.

17. Black, M. M., & Aboud, F. E. (2011). Responsive feeding is embedded in a theoretical framework of responsive parenting. *Journal of Nutrition, 141*(3), 490–494. doi:10.3945/jn.110.129973.

18. Sinha, R. (2018). Role of addiction and stress neurobiology on food intake and obesity. *Biological Psychology, 131,* 5–13. doi:10.1016/j.biopsycho.2017.05.001.

19. Yeung, A. Y., & Tadi, P. (2023). *Physiology, obesity neurohormonal appetite and satiety control.* StatPearls. https://www.ncbi.nlm.nih.gov/books/NBK555906/

20. Michaelsen, K. F., Grummer-Strawn, L., & Bégin, F. (2017). Emerging issues in complementary feeding: Global aspects. *Maternal & Child Nutrition, 13*(Suppl 2), Article e12444. doi:10.1111/mcn.12444.

21. Carnell, S., Thapaliya, G., Jansen, E., et al. (2023). Biobehavioral susceptibility for obesity in childhood: Behavioral, genetic and neuroimaging studies of appetite. *Physiology & Behavior, 271,* 114313. doi:10.1016/j.physbeh.2023.114313.

22. Scaglioni, S., De Cosmi, V., Ciappolino, V., et al. (2018). Factors influencing children's eating behaviours. *Nutrients, 10*(6), 706. doi:10.3390/nu10060706.

23. Tylka, T. L., Lumeng, J. C., & Eneli, I. U. (2015). Maternal intuitive eating as a moderator of the association between concern about child weight and restrictive child feeding. *Appetite, 95,* 158–165. doi:10.1016/j.appet.2015.06.023.

24. Savage, J. S., Fisher, J. O., & Birch, L. L. (2007). Parental influence on eating behavior: Conception to adolescence. *Journal of Law, Medicine & Ethics, 35*(1), 22–34. doi:10.1111/j.1748-720X.2007.00111.x.

25. Øverby, N. C., Hillesund, E. R., Røed, M., et al. (2020). Association between parental feeding practices and shared family meals. The Food4toddlers study. *Food & Nutrition Research, 64.* doi:10.29219/fnr.v64.4456.

26. Fildes, A., van Jaarsveld, C. H., Llewellyn, C., et al. (2015). Parental control over feeding in infancy. Influence of infant weight, appetite and feeding method. *Appetite, 91,* 101–106. doi:10.1016/j.appet.2015.04.004.

27. Carper, J. L., Orlet Fisher, J., & Birch, L. L. (2000). Young girls' emerging dietary restraint and disinhibition are related to parental control in child feeding. *Appetite, 35*(2), 121–129. doi:10.1006/appe.2000.0343.

28. Jensen, M. L., Dillman Carpentier, F. R., Corvalán, C., et al. (2022). Television viewing and using screens while eating: Associations with dietary intake in children and adolescents. *Appetite, 168,* 105670. doi:10.1016/j.appet.2021.105670.

29. Eli, K., Howell, K., Fisher, P. A., et al. (2014). "Those comments last forever": Parents and grandparents of preschoolers recount how they became aware of their own body weights as children. *PLoS One, 9*(11), Article e111974. doi:10.1371/journal.pone.0111974.

30. World Health Organization. (2023). WHO Guideline for complementary

feeding of infants and young children 6–23 months of age. https://www.ncbi
.nlm.nih.gov/books/NBK596427/

31. Patel, J. K., & Rouster, A. S. (2022). *Infant nutrition requirements and options.*
StatPearls. https://www.ncbi.nlm.nih.gov/books/NBK560758/

32. Patel, J. K., & Rouster, A. S. (2022).

33. World Health Organization. (2017). *Nutritional anaemias: tools for effective
prevention and control.* https://www.who.int/publications/i/item/9789241513067

34. Daniels, L., Taylor, R. W., Williams, S. M., et al. (2018). Impact of a modified
version of baby-led weaning on iron intake and status: A randomised
controlled trial. *BMJ Open, 8*(6), Article e019036. doi:10.1136/bmjopen-2017
-019036.

35. Martinez-Torres, V., Torres, N., Davis, J. A., et al. (2023). Anemia and associated
risk factors in pediatric patients. *Pediatric Health, Medicine & Therapeutics, 14,*
267–280. doi:10.2147/PHMT.S389105.

36. Graczykowska, K., Kaczmarek, J., Wilczyńska, D., et al. (2021). The
consequence of excessive consumption of cow's milk: Protein-losing
enteropathy with anasarca in the course of iron deficiency anemia-case reports
and a literature review. *Nutrients, 13*(3), 828. doi:10.3390/nu13030828.

37. United States Food & Drug Administration. (2024). *Arsenic in Food.* https://
www.fda.gov/food/environmental-contaminants-food/arsenic-food

38. United States Food & Drug Administration. (2022). *What You Can Do to Limit
Exposure to Arsenic.* https://www.fda.gov/food/environmental-contaminants
-food/arsenic-food

39. United States Food & Drug Administration. (2022). *What You Can Do to
Limit Exposure to Arsenic and Lead in Fruit Juices.* https://www.fda.gov/food/
environmental-contaminants-food/what-you-can-do-limit-exposure-arsenic
-and-lead-juices

40. United States Food & Drug Administration. (2023). *Help Protect Children from
Environmental Contaminants: Healthy Food Choices for Your Baby Aged 6 to 12 Months.*
https://www.fda.gov/food/environmental-contaminants-food/help-protect
-children-environmental-contaminants-healthy-food-choices-your-baby-aged
-6-12-months

41. United States Food & Drug Administration. (2024). *Mercury in Food.* https://
www.fda.gov/food/environmental-contaminants-food/mercury-food

42. Emmerik, N. E., de Jong, F., & van Elburg, R. M. (2020). Dietary intake of
sodium during infancy and the cardiovascular consequences later in life: A
scoping review. *Annals of Nutrition & Metabolism, 76*(2), 114–121. doi.org/
10.1159/000507354.

43. Scaglioni, S., De Cosmi, V., Ciappolino, V., et al. (2018). Factors influencing
children's eating behaviours. *Nutrients, 10*(6), 706.

44. Yang, S. & Wang, H. (2023). Avoidance of added salt for 6–12-month-old
infants: A narrative review. *Archives de Pédiatrie.*

45. Strazzullo, P., Campanozzi, A., & Avallone, S. (2012). Does salt intake in the
first two years of life affect the development of cardiovascular disorders in
adulthood? *Nutrition, Metabolism and Cardiovascular Diseases, 22*(10),
787–792. doi:10.1016/j.numecd.2012.04.003.

46. Liem, D. G. (2017). Infants' and children's salt taste perception and liking: A review. *Nutrients, 9*(9), 1011.
47. Jansen, E., Mulkens, S., Emond, Y., & Jansen, A. (2008). From the Garden of Eden to the land of plenty: Restriction of fruit and sweets intake leads to increased fruit and sweets consumption in children. *Appetite, 51*(3), 570–575. doi:10.1016/j.appet.2008.04.012.
48. Tylka, T. L., Lumeng, J. C., & Eneli, I. U. (2015). Maternal intuitive eating as a moderator of the association between concern about child weight and restrictive child feeding. *Appetite, 95,* 158–165.
49. Fildes, A., van Jaarsveld, C. H., & Llewellyn, C., et al. (2015). Parental control over feeding in infancy. Influence of infant weight, appetite and feeding method. *Appetite, 91,* 101–106.
50. Carper, J. L., Fisher, J. O., & Birch, L. L. (2000). Young girls' emerging dietary restraint and disinhibition are related to parental control in child feeding. *Appetite, 35*(2), 121–129. doi:10.1006/appe.2000.0343.
51. Johannsen, D. L., Johannsen, N. M., & Specker, B. L. (2006). Influence of parents' eating behaviors and child feeding practices on children's weight status. *Obesity, 14*(3), 431–439. doi:10.1038/oby.2006.57.
52. Heyman, M. B., Abrams, S. A., Heitlinger, L. A., et al. (2017). Fruit juice in infants, children, and adolescents: Current recommendations. *Pediatrics, 139*(6). doi:10.1542/peds.2017-0967.
53. Park, S., Lin, M., Onufrak, S., & Li, R. (2015). Association of sugar-sweetened beverage intake during infancy with dental caries in 6-year-olds. *Clinical Nutrition Research, 4*(1), 9.
54. Øverby, N. C., Hillesund, E. R., Røed, M., et al. (2020). Association between parental feeding practices and shared family meals. The Food4toddlers study. *Food & Nutrition Research, 64.* doi:10.29219/fnr.v64.4456.
55. Emmerik, N. E., de Jong, F., & van Elburg, R. M. (2020). Dietary intake of sodium during infancy and the cardiovascular consequences later in life: A Scoping Review. *Annals of Nutrition & Metabolism, 76*(2), 114–121. doi.org/10.1159/000507354.
56. Scaglioni, S., De Cosmi, V., Ciappolino, V., et al. (2018). Factors influencing children's eating behaviours. *Nutrients, 10*(6), 706.
57. Øverby, N. C., Hillesund, E. R., Røed, M., et al. (2020).
58. Garza, C., & de Onis M. (2004). Rationale for developing a new international growth reference. *Food & Nutrition Bulletin, 25*(Suppl 1), S5–S14. doi:10.1177/15648265040251S102.

Chapter Sixteen

1. Arvedson, J. C., Brodsky, L., and Lefton-Greif, M. (2019). *Pediatric swallowing and feeding: Assessment and management* (3rd ed). Plural.
2. Singleton, N., and Shulman, B. (2014). *Language development: Foundations, processes, and clinical applications* (2nd ed). Jones & Bartlett Learning.
3. Del Rosario, C., Slevin, M., Molloy, E. J., et al. (2021). How to use the Bayley scales of infant and toddler development. *Archives of Disease in Childhood-Education and Practice, 106*(2), 108–112.

4.   Bayley, N. (2006). Bayley scales of infant and toddler development. Psychological Corporation. [Bayley Scales of Infant and Toddler Development is a formal assessment tool for diagnosing developmental delays in childhood.]

5.   Madigan, S., Prime, H., Graham, S. A., et al. (2019). Parenting behavior and child language: A meta-analysis. *Pediatrics, 144*(4), Article e20183556. doi:10.1542/peds.2018-3556.

6.   Weisleder, A., & Fernald, A. (2013). Talking to children matters: Early language experience strengthens processing and builds vocabulary. *Psychological Science, 24*(11), 2143–2152. doi:10.1177/0956797613488145.

Chapter Seventeen

1.   Bayley, N. (2006). Bayley scales of infant and toddler development. Psychological Corporation. [Bayley Scales of Infant and Toddler Development is a formal assessment tool for diagnosing developmental delays in childhood.]

2.   Arvedson J. C., Brodsky L., & Lefton-Greif, M. (2019). *Pediatric swallowing and feeding: Assessment and management* (3rd ed). Plural.

3.   Singleton, N., & Shulman, B. (2014). *Language development: Foundations, processes, and clinical applications* (2nd ed). Jones & Bartlett Learning.

4.   Del Rosario, C., Slevin, M., Molloy, E. J., et al. (2021). How to use the Bayley scales of infant and toddler development. *Archives of Disease in Childhood- Education and Practice, 106*(2), 108–112.

Chapter Eighteen

1.   Bayley, N. (2006). Bayley scales of infant and toddler development. Psychological Corporation. [Bayley Scales of Infant and Toddler Development is a formal assessment tool for diagnosing developmental delays in childhood.]

2.   Arvedson, J. C., Brodsky, L., & Lefton-Greif, M. (2019). *Pediatric swallowing and feeding: Assessment and management* (3rd ed). Plural.

3.   Singleton, N., & Shulman, B. (2014). *Language development: Foundations, processes, and clinical applications.* (2nd ed). Jones & Bartlett Learning.

4.   Del Rosario, C., Slevin, M., Molloy, E. J., et al. (2021). How to use the Bayley scales of infant and toddler development. *Archives of Disease in Childhood- Education and Practice, 106*(2), 108–112.

Chapter Nineteen

1.   Bayley, N. (2006). Bayley scales of infant and toddler development. Psychological Corporation. [Bayley Scales of Infant and Toddler Development is a formal assessment tool for diagnosing developmental delays in childhood.]

2.   Arvedson, J. C., Brodsky, L., & Lefton-Greif, M. (2019). *Pediatric swallowing and feeding: Assessment and management* (3rd ed). Plural.

3.   Del Rosario, C., Slevin, M., Molloy, E. J., et al. (2021). How to use the Bayley scales of infant and toddler development. *Archives of Disease in Childhood- Education and Practice, 106*(2), 108–112.

4.   Arvedson, J. C., Brodsky, L., & Lefton-Greif, M. (2019).

5.   Singleton, N., & Shulman, B. (2014). *Language development: Foundations, processes, and clinical applications.* (2nd ed). Jones & Bartlett Learning.

6. Meek, J. Y., Noble, L., & Section on Breastfeeding. (2022). Policy statement: breastfeeding and the use of human milk. *Pediatrics, 150*(1), e2022057988.

Problem Solving

1. Tabbers, M. M., DiLorenzo, C., Berger, M. Y., et al. (2014). Evaluation and treatment of functional constipation in infants and children: Evidence-based recommendations from ESPGHAN and NASPGHAN. *Journal of Pediatric Gastroenterology & Nutrition, 58*(2), 258–274. doi:10.1097/MPG.0000000000000266.
2. Tabbers, M. M., DiLorenzo, C., Berger, M. Y., et al. (2014). Evaluation and treatment of functional constipation in infants and children: Evidence-based recommendations from ESPGHAN and NASPGHAN. *Journal of Pediatric Gastroenterology & Nutrition, 58*(2), 258–274. doi:10.1097/MPG.0000000000000266.
3. National Institutes of Health. (2020). *Symptoms & causes of GER & GERD in infants.* National Institute of Diabetes and Digestive and Kidney Diseases. https://www.niddk.nih.gov/health-information/digestive-diseases/acid-reflux-ger-gerd-infants/symptoms-causes
4. GI Kids. (n.d.). *GERD & reflux in infants.* https://gikids.org/gerd/gerd-infants/

Resources for Families with Allergies

1. Weir, W. B., Fred, L. Y., Pike, M., et al. (2018). Expired epinephrine maintains chemical concentration and sterility. *Prehospital Emergency Care, 22*(4), 414–418. doi:10.1080/10903127.2017.1402109.
2. Simons, F. E., Gu, X., & Simons, K. J. (2000). Outdated EpiPen and EpiPen Jr autoinjectors: Past their prime? *Journal of Allergy & Clinical Immunology, 105*(5) 1025–1030. doi:10.1067/mai.2000.106042.
3. Rachid, O., Simons, F. E., Wein, M. B., et al. (2015). Epinephrine doses contained in outdated epinephrine auto-injectors collected in a Florida allergy practice. *Annals of Allergy, Asthma & Immunology, 114*(4), 354–356.e1. doi:10.1016/j.anai.2015.01.015.

Index

Let's keep a good thing going!

Scan the code to stay connected,
explore more tips, and get special offers
on our app and other resources.

SolidStarts.com